A ... sed
b ... ought *with* Good
Manners, a biography of Margaret Rutherford, *Greasepaint and Cordite: How ENSA Entertained the Troops During World War II*, and *A Minor Adjustment*, his earlier book about becoming the parent of a child with Down's Syndrome. He also co-wrote *Killa*, the autobiography of the Republic of Ireland footballer and TV pundit Kevin Kilbane, and contributed to Peter Davison's memoir, *Is There Life Outside the Box?* He and his family live in north London.

All royalties from this book go to the
Down's Syndrome Association, www.downs-syndrome.org.uk

A Major Adjustment

How a Remarkable Child Became a Remarkable Adult

Andy Merriman

Foreword by Michel Roux Jr

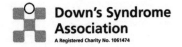

Down's Syndrome Association
A Registered Charity No. 1061474

First published 2018 by
The Down's Syndrome Association
Langdon Down Centre
2a Langdon Park
Teddington
Middlesex
TW11 9PS
www.downs-syndrome.org.uk

Typeset in Sabon and Mr Eaves by SX Composing DTP, Rayleigh, Essex
Printed and bound in the UK by Clays Ltd, St Ives plc

This book is in memory of Sarah's beloved grandfathers:

ERIC MERRIMAN ('Grandpa Eric')
and
JOHN WELLEMIN ('Pop John')

Contents

Foreword

When I was first approached by Channel 4 to present a pro-gramme taking on the issues that people with disabilities face when finding employment, I immediately knew that this was something I wanted and had to do. I take on as much charitable work as I possibly can and, I have to admit, it leaves me frustrated when I have to decline helping good causes. *Kitchen Impossible*, as the series came to be called, turned out to be an incredible rev-elation for me: to be part of such a thought-provoking emotional rollercoaster, and to get to meet and work with these incredible individuals, was indeed an honour.

Nothing could have prepared me for the first day of filming. I consider myself strong of character and capable of dealing with most situations, but witnessing an hour long 'tic' attack from one of the contributors who had Tourette's syndrome, and not knowing what to do or say, was something I had never experienced. Soon after, I tasted a perfect omelette cooked by another contributor, a blind chef, and these were just two of the moments that will stay with me forever.

A Major Adjustment

Not knowing how to react, no longer trusting my instincts, afraid to offend, and wanting to be more charitable, were just a few of the emotions I had during that first day. I found myself addressing the group as though they were children rather than adults, helping them to do simple tasks when I should have been talking to and treating them as equals, not helping or feeling sorry for them, but challenging them. But the experience was eye-opening – soon enough I had realised that being charitable and nice was not going to get us anywhere, so I set about looking for the ability, not the disability, and I found it by the bucketload.

Amongst the group of people taking part was a young lady with Down's Syndrome called Sarah. What was immediately evident was how driven Sarah is, with a very clear vision of what she wanted to achieve, but also how she always has time for others, and is a real team player. Often, Sarah could be found encouraging the others and challenging them to do better; at times she even took the lead in tasks.

Her dream was to be a barista, and nothing was going to get in her way, and finally she got her chance, in an Italian restaurant that we took over for the show. To see Sarah standing by her espresso machine with such pride was a joy. I don't think I have ever drunk so much coffee in my life!

Finding jobs for any one of the group was never going to be easy, and although that was the aim of the programme and the 'holy grail', there were other things that were equally as important: changing general perceptions, discovering and nurturing ability, being accepted for who you are and, ultimately, not being defined by your disability.

It fills me with pride that in a very small way I have helped Sarah and the others achieve their potential. I absolutely loved

Foreword

working with the group, and am so happy with the result. I miss the camaraderie and friendship that evolved during the filming – it was an experience I will always treasure. I'm so glad she is doing so well. For me it was never in doubt, as she is a star!

Michel Roux Jr

Prologue

I rang my daughter in enthusiastic mode, and told her that there was going to be another book about her. Sarah was excited. 'Great! Don't forget – I'm going to write it.'

'Ahh. . .' I recalled the last paragraph of *A Minor Adjustment*, which I had published in 1999, about my experience of becoming the parent of a child with Down's Syndrome. 'Sarah,' I had written,

> you've been my inspiration in so many ways – least of all you've been my muse. So, if you're reading this and you want to continue to be my goddess of divine influence, now that I've finished the book, I'm looking for work. Oh, no, that's no good, I'm definitely not going to write another book about you. Absolutely not. You see, if there's going to be a sequel in years to come . . . I want you to write it.

Hmm. . . I was bit stymied. 'Well, we need to think about it.'

'How come I'm not writing this book?' Sarah persisted. 'You promised!'

Prologue

'Well, you were only six when I said that. And I didn't really ever think you could . . . and it's very complicated, writing a book.'

'Tell me about it,' said Sarah.

'Exactly!'

'But I can do it. I'm twenty-five now.'

'Well. . . OK: how about we write some of it together? How does that sound?'

'Good idea!'

'When should we meet? What are you up to this week?'

'Don't know – I'm a bit busy at the moment. . .'

'OK – shall I make a start?'

'Good idea, Dad.'

'And I want you to begin writing as well.'

'OK, Dad. I'll let you go now. Love you. Bye!'

A few months later, I was still awaiting a contribution, although I did receive a text from Sarah which read, 'I love you dad how is our book doing?'

Fortunately, I have been able to include many contributions from Sarah, mainly from cards, speeches, messages and texts she has written over the years. They are reproduced as originally written, and spelling or grammar mistakes have not been corrected – so no blame is attached to my editor!

For reasons of brevity, I have occasionally shortened 'Down's syndrome' to 'Down's or 'DS', but this is clearly not intended as a diminution of the condition. These are also terms that our family use informally.

1

A MINOR ADJUSTMENT

Without deviation from the norm, progress is not possible.

Frank Zappa

The lyrics of Cole Porter's seminal love song 'Ev'ry Time We Say Goodbye' contain these words:

> There's no love song finer,
> But how strange the change,
> From major to minor,
> Ev'ry time we say goodbye.

Although I may not 'die a little' every time I say goodbye to Sarah, I do miss her when she's not around. Her presence is comforting, reassuring and inspiring. As her older brother Daniel once remarked, 'Sarah is the heartbeat of the family.' In the key of life Sarah has now made the change from minor to major . . .

About ten years ago, we were attending a Down's Syndrome Association Christmas carol concert as a family when a woman tapped me on the shoulder. She had undergone pre-natal testing, she told me, and discovered she was expecting a baby with Down's syndrome. So while she had been pregnant, she had read *A Minor Adjustment*.

That was a very brave thing to do, I told her: parts of the book were brutally honest about having a child with a disability.

She replied that she had been in some torment about whether to have the baby or terminate her pregnancy.

So what had she decided, I asked?

She pointed to a young girl: 'That's Beth. I read your book, and I thought it would be fine. . .'

It was an incredibly emotional moment; one I will never forget.

When I was first approached back in 1997 to write Sarah's story, in what was to become *A Minor Adjustment*, I was somewhat daunted by the enormity of the task. Not only was it going to be a lot of work but, more pertinently, it would also have to chart the first few years of Sarah's life in a stark and truthful manner, which would inevitably involve much breast-beating and soul-baring. My wife, Alison (Allie), was excited by the prospect, but was also naturally apprehensive. The only person amongst my immediate circle who was absolutely certain about the project was Sarah herself. But then that's Sarah. One hundred per cent enthusiastic.

As in *A Minor Adjustment*, which told the story of Sarah's life from her birth until the age of five, this book is primarily about Sarah, and how she fits into our story thus far. I don't, however, mean to suggest that she is a representative of everyone with Down's syndrome, because people with the syndrome are all individuals with their own characters and idiosyncrasies. We are also lucky that Sarah has enjoyed good health, and I am also aware that many parents reading this will have children who suffer from serious health problems, or have dual diagnoses that can cause additional developmental delay. There are parents who are still striving for the basic educational rights, and those whose children might never be able to achieve any kind of independence – even if given the opportunity. It is easy to become self-satisfied when I think of Sarah and how much she has done, but we must not forget that for some people having a child with disabilities can be extremely challenging – no matter what support, opportunities or resources are available.

A Minor Adjustment was published in 1999 to much interest and publicity, with articles in the national press prompting interviews and appearances on several national television shows. The book was best summed up by the novelist and academic David Lodge, himself the father of a son with Down's:

> *A Minor Adjustment* is a warm but completely unsentimental account of the experience of parenting a Down's child, with some broader reflections on the nature and social history of the condition. It is written clearly and honestly (sometimes painfully so), with love and a delightful sense of humour. Parents who are facing the same challenge will find this book both encouraging and useful.

The impact of the book went far beyond my expectations. The paperback edition was distributed by health professionals to new parents of babies with Down's syndrome, and reached a wider audience when serialised in two national newspapers, the *Daily Mail* and the *Guardian* – while the positive reaction from other parents to the book's candour was overwhelming. I was told of one couple who had had a baby with Down's syndrome, and decided that they couldn't keep her and would put her up for adoption. Their social worker suggested they read Sarah's book first. They did – and decided to change their decision and keep their daughter.

It's now nearly twenty years since *A Minor Adjustment* was published, which is why it's time to tell the next stage of Sarah's story: of how that little girl grew up into a young woman and made her way out into the world. Many new readers will not have had the opportunity to read the first book, while those that did will no doubt not mind having their memories refreshed, so I'll happily confess that most of the rest of this and the next chapter, and several parts of forthcoming chapters, are largely reproduced from *Minor*. It was Alfred Hitchcock who is quoted as having declared that 'Self-plagiarism is style.' He should know . . . although I would like to state that no blondes were harmed in the writing of this book.

A Minor Adjustment itself would not have happened had the book's publishers not been intrigued and charmed by a comedy drama series on BBC Radio 4 called *Minor Adjustment*. The series told the story of a family and their four-year-old child with Down's syndrome, and starred Peter Davison, Samantha Bond and . . . Sarah Merriman. The idea for the drama came from me and my father, Sarah's grandfather, Eric Merriman, whose distinguished comedy scriptwriting career included *Beyond Our Ken,* and we wrote it together. The cast members had been extremely patient and kind to Sarah, and her presence added an authenticity to the family drama. She performed and behaved beautifully, and I couldn't have been more proud of her. 'No, this wasn't how the script was supposed to read' seemed an adroit, if inadvertent description of Sarah's life thus far.

On Sarah's original debut at the Whittington Hospital's labour ward on 9 January 1992, however, we certainly did not feel that 'A star was born'. There had been no reason to believe that the birth of our second child was going to be much different from that of our first two years earlier. Although he was nearly two weeks late and the labour was long and tortuous, the arrival of Daniel, our first-born, had been fairly straightforward. Well, it was certainly straightforward for me – I just watched. It was slightly more arduous for Allie, although I have to say she went through the whole process without even an aspirin.

Being of the liberal persuasion and also living in north London, it was apparently mandatory that we attend the local Natural Childbirth Trust group, and so we did have some idea of what was supposed to happen. Fortunately our particular group had been informative without being precious – there wasn't a beanbag in sight, and none of the men felt envious or guilty about not being able to breastfeed. Of course, I did have to explain to Allie that 'natural childbirth' didn't mean giving birth without wearing make-up.

Daniel had been born at the Whittington Hospital where both Allie and I had worked as social workers, and when Allie became pregnant with Sarah she remained under the care of the same consultant obstetrician. There weren't any problems during the pregnancy and, apart from the usual scans, which all appeared to be normal, Allie also had the Alfa Feta Protein blood test, which gives an approximate idea of any possible birth defects. The results did not show anything unusual.

The night before Sarah was born, we were watching a Paul Simon concert on television, and he sang a song called 'Born at the Wrong Time'. Allie had already started to go into labour, and we both remarked that, as it was likely the baby would now be born in the middle of the night, these words seemed somewhat prophetic. I was being flippant, but Allie said later that, to her surprise, this song had filled her with panic and a sense of foreboding.

As Allie's contractions grew stronger, I rang my mother, who had arranged to come and stay and look after Daniel. As soon as she arrived we sped to the hospital, which was only about fifteen minutes away. After an initial examination, the process seemed to slow down, and at about two o'clock in the morning it was decided that I could go home, but Allie should remain in hospital. By the time I reached the labour ward at about nine o'clock the next morning Allie was having regular and painful contractions and, although the moment of delivery was obviously imminent, I would be present and politically correct at the birth.

At 9.45 a.m. our baby arrived as if propelled from a huge gun – a human cannonball who seemed to fly through the air into the safe arms of one of the two midwives in attendance. It was a girl, just as we had wanted: our luck had held out again. We now had a boy and a girl. 'It's my dream come true,' said Allie.

Sarah was quite blue, and seemed to be struggling for air. The first thing I said to Allie was, 'She looks like a little Buddha.' Sarah was put into an incubator, and very soon her colour became a more healthy-looking pink. I went off to telephone both sets of grandparents and inform them that all was well, and that their first granddaughter had arrived safe and sound.

Whilst I was away, Allie was naturally engrossed with her new-born child, and studied every detail. She seemed perfect in every way, and her expression even displayed a curiously independent air. But the longer this loving examination continued, the more Allie started to feel something was wrong. She looked more carefully at Sarah's face, and noticed a number of particular features she had seen in some other children. Sarah had small, protruding ears, a round face and a wide bridge of the nose. An ominous image began to form in her mind.

Desperately trying to remember other characteristics, Allie checked for more signs. There was a large gap between Sarah's big toe and the rest of her toes, and her fingers were short and stubby. Allie took Sarah's hand and searched for the palmic crease, but couldn't see a significant line. But Sarah's weight had been above-average, and she was already starting to breastfeed – perhaps, in the aftermath of giving birth and the ensuing sense of unreality, Allie's imagination had taken over?

Confused, her mind in a whirl, Allie told the midwife she thought Sarah's features corresponded with those of Down's syndrome, hoping for some reassurance along the lines of, 'Oh, all babies look a bit funny and squashed when they're born.'

Frighteningly, the midwife's response was, 'I'd better call the paediatrician.'

I returned to the delivery room ten minutes later, and Allie told me what had happened. I looked to the midwife for some instant reassurance, but she was busying herself with cleaning up, and clearly too engrossed to confirm or deny.

During the birth, Allie had been torn, and was now being stitched. She seemed not to notice the pain – could only stare at Sarah, hoping that all was well. I took Sarah out of her cot, held her in my arms, and stared at her.

It was immediately apparent: she did indeed have Down's syndrome. How could I not have noticed the obvious features the moment she was born? Her eyes were almond-shaped, her neck was short and thick, and the back of her head seemed somewhat flat.

'What do you think?' asked Allie.

'I don't know,' I said. 'It's too difficult to tell.'

'She's very floppy, isn't she?'

'So would you be if you'd just been born,' I said weakly.

We both knew the reality, but felt too helpless to confront the truth. Whilst Allie was still receiving medical attention I felt I had to be comforting and optimistic.

A Minor Adjustment

After what seemed like an eternity, but was actually only about fifteen minutes, the consultant paediatrician arrived with a junior doctor. We both knew Dr Mackinnon well as we had worked with her. I sat on the bed holding Allie's hand, and both doctors examined Sarah.

Dr Mackinnon finished her examination, and turned to us, nodding. Yes, she said, she did think Sarah had Down's syndrome. She apologised, as though she herself bore some fault or blame, and hugged us both. The diagnosis would have to be confirmed by a blood test, she said, and we should have the results within a week. There was just a very slight chance that the diagnosis would not be confirmed, but we all knew there would be no reprieve. Dr Mackinnon offered us some kind words and said she thought we should be left alone to talk, but that she would come back later. She and her colleagues left us on our own. I picked Sarah up and held her closely in my arms. 'Oh, Sarah, Sarah,' I whispered to her, 'what have you done? You've got it all wrong. . .'

Allie and I cried together, and my thoughts turned to the adults with Down's syndrome I had worked with as a social worker nearly 20 years earlier. The image that had always stuck in my mind was that of middle-aged women with hair in ribbons, attired like little girls in ill-fitting dresses, drab cardigans and white, knee-high socks. People like this were supposed to be clients of mine – people I was employed to help – not my own daughter, who was supposed to be bright and beautiful. These people attended adult training centres for 'the handicapped', performing menial tasks for little pleasure or reward. My daughter was going to go to university and become a doctor or a barrister. People with Down's syndrome were patronised, joked about and exploited, and still referred to as 'mongols'.

This was not how it was supposed to be.

A Major Adjustment

I went to phone the grandparents – only this time to tell them that the news wasn't so good. Allie's parents had gone out, so I spoke to her sister, Carey. She could barely believe what I told her. She said she would talk to her parents, and I was somewhat grateful that I now wouldn't have to. I rang my parents again, and this time talked to my mother. She is an extremely stoical person, and to my relief, because I really felt too distressed to discuss it, she took the news calmly, barely commenting. She would tell my dad, she said, for which I was equally grateful.

Back on the labour ward, two close friends, Pat and Annie, who had also worked in the hospital with us, had arrived to see Allie. They looked pale and shocked, and I started to cry as soon as I saw them. We all embraced, and none of us knew quite what to say. We had asked Annie to be Sarah's godmother, and the only thing I could think of to ask was whether Sarah having Down's syndrome would make any difference – whether Annie would still want to be godmother, which of course she did! If our new baby was a girl we had always planned to call her Sarah, but soon afterwards Allie and I even found ourselves discussing whether we should still call the baby Sarah, as now she was going to be so patently different from the new daughter we had originally pictured.

After Pat and Annie had left, we talked to one of the midwives who had delivered Sarah, and it emerged that she had a 30-year-old brother who had Down's syndrome. He was studying accountancy, she told us, he had a girlfriend, and he was leading a pretty full life. She was the very first person of many who, over the years to come, would give us encouraging examples of friends or relatives with Down's syndrome.

Although we were still in a state of shock, it was important to hear something so positive. Even at the time I thought how much of a coincidence it was that, from the moment of birth, Sarah had a link with another person who had Down's syndrome.

When we were left on our own once again, we tried to make some sense of it all. 'We are going to keep her, aren't we?' asked Allie.

Without thinking, I replied, 'Of course we are.' At that stage I seriously hadn't considered any other option, but it transpired that Allie was thinking of clients of hers, a couple who had had a baby with Down's syndrome and not kept the child: the husband had refused to accept the baby's condition, and the wife had been put in the impossible position of choosing between her husband and her child. She chose the husband, and the baby was adopted.

Even a couple of hours after Sarah's birth, we were both quite clear that we wanted to take her home. There didn't seem to be any realistic alternative, but it was actually very helpful when the consultant obstetrician, Miss Morgan, came to see us. As social workers and supposedly responsible people, who had counselled others in the very position we now found ourselves in, she told us, we would feel we just had to cope, and there would be an assumption that we would just get on with it. But if Sarah's arrival was too much to bear, she made it clear – if we felt under too much pressure to manage – we should consider having her fostered, to give us time to think about the future. Although we both knew from our work that this was an option, it was very important for it to be spelled out to us so clearly. We did have an obligation to Sarah, but we also had a responsibility to Daniel and to one another. Sarah was now part of our family, but not at any cost.

Later that morning, Allie and Sarah were transferred to a post-natal ward. Fortunately they were allocated a room to themselves, so at least we would have some privacy. By this time I really had had enough: I couldn't wait to get away from the hospital, and even from Allie, as I no longer knew what to say to her. The strain of being the main source of support was beginning to affect me, and my words of reassurance now sounded hollow. It had been agreed that I would collect Daniel from his childminder and bring him back to the hospital to meet his new sibling as soon as possible: here was my chance to escape!

But while before the birth we had all got very excited at the prospect of Daniel's reaction, now I couldn't bear the thought of seeing him. Although he was only two years and three months and obviously wouldn't understand all the implications of Sarah's birth, he would be able to gauge my mood soon enough. When Daniel had been born, I couldn't wait to go into the nearest toyshop and celebrate by buying him the inevitable teddy bear. This time was different. I felt numb and distressed, and certainly not in the mood for bounding into a shop and excitedly choosing something for Sarah. Although I knew I was already letting Sarah down, I just couldn't face buying her a present. It didn't seem like a time to celebrate anything. This trip to the childminder had become horribly daunting. Thankfully, Annie took charge and insisted on driving me to collect Daniel, and on the way she bought a wonderful teddy bear for Sarah.

Annie had telephoned ahead to tell the childminder what had happened. As a former nursing sister at Great Ormond Street Hospital for Children she was quite used to drama and crises, and when we got there she was extremely sympathetic and calm. I went into the room where Daniel was playing and as soon as I saw him I broke down in tears. This wasn't the sister he was supposed to have – and would he now have to be responsible for her for the rest of his life? I told him he had a baby sister and, although he had said he wanted a brother, he seemed happy enough. Amazingly, he didn't seem to notice my anguish, but I was already wondering how and when we would tell him about Sarah – at the moment he was obviously too young to understand, but how soon would he realise that something was wrong?

Annie drove Daniel and me back to the hospital, where my mother and Allie's parents had now arrived. No one quite knew what to say, but everybody was trying to make it as 'normal' as possible, whilst acknowledging the reality of the situation. One of the nurses popped in to say that Sarah was due to have a scan – as it is common for children with Down's syndrome to have heart defects, we had been warned soon after Sarah's birth that she would need one. I quickly volunteered to take her, as I was finding it very difficult to face the family without breaking down.

I thus found myself pushing a large, transparent hospital cot containing my tiny daughter around the very same corridors where I had worked for nearly ten years. Inevitably, on the way I met quite a few colleagues and acquaintances, all of whom were interested in my new daughter, but all of whom I wanted to keep at a distance and not have to explain what had happened. In the Special Care Baby Unit another consultant paediatrician was waiting for us, and we walked past the half-dozen incubators containing babies of minute size – one or two as small as my hand – to be shown into a side room.

As the various clouds and fuzzy images appeared on the screen, I looked down at this tiny creature and felt very little for her other than sympathy that she had to start her life in such disastrous circumstances. Perhaps, if she did have an inoperable heart condition, it might be so serious that she might not survive for very long. Perhaps, if it was serious, she might have to undergo major surgery on more than one occasion. Perhaps, if she was not going to have any quality of life – a future of poor health and a severe learning disability – then it might be better for everyone, and especially her, if she just passed away. . . I was looking at my daughter – not even a day old – and wishing her dead.

A couple of days after her birth, Sarah was ready to leave hospital. She was still quite jaundiced, but it was agreed that, if we kept a careful check on her, she would be able to come home. We departed quietly, with a few words of thanks to the ward staff, but desperately not wanting a fuss or a big goodbye. It was a relief to be out of the hospital, and leave behind the constant labelling that had marked her arrival. 'What have you got – a boy or a girl?'

'Actually . . . it's a Down's syndrome baby.'

It was as if Sarah did not have an identity of her own, and wasn't really our baby. She belonged to another extended family, chromosomal cousins called 'the Downses', with their own physical characteristics, their own lifestyle and their own culture. We had somehow unexpectedly inherited this baby from them, but were now expected to raise her as one of our own. She had little hair, and what she did have was blonde. She was round-faced, snub-nosed and almond-eyed. She didn't look like us. She was certainly very different from Daniel – with his shock of black hair and familial facial features, unmistakably a product of his parents' genes. But this one, well, she didn't really seem to be one of the Merrimans, and yet here she was, and was now expected to come and live in our house. Perhaps she was just a lodger who wouldn't be staying long – maybe she wouldn't fit in with us, and would have to be returned to whence she came.

It was a very subdued homecoming, and we really didn't quite know how to behave. It was a bit like New Year's Eve when you know the approaching year is going to be difficult. The event had to be marked – but in what way? We were in no mood for celebrating, and yet here was our newborn baby coming home for the first time. We smuggled her in through the front door as quickly as possible so that the neighbours wouldn't see her, and we would all be saved from any difficult doorstep conversations and embarrassing moments.

I had put up a 'WELCOME HOME, SARAH AND MUMMY' paper banner in the hallway, which I had hastily made the previous day. I was not known for my decorative artwork, and now, suspended at an oblique angle having partly freed itself from the wall, it appeared even more forlorn and tatty. The house was so full of tulips, daffodils and carnations that Allie remarked that it resembled a funeral parlour. 'Say it with flowers', is how the slogan reads, but what was the 'it' that friends and family were trying to say?

The first few weeks after Sarah's homecoming were filled with a regular procession of people, all bearing gifts and helping in every way possible. Between them, friends delivered meals, did the shopping, took Daniel off our hands for a few hours to play, and one neighbour even arranged for him to attend her son's playgroup, pushing a double buggy up a steep hill three days a week. Not only did the immediate family rally round, but friends of friends appeared or telephoned with offers of all sorts of help. A week's supply of home-cooked meals was delivered by an old friend of Allie's, and there were many invitations from others, providing understanding, sustenance and good counsel. Friends from all over Britain made the effort to come and see us, and we also had a visit from our Dutch friends Frank and Christine, who actually made a day trip from the Netherlands. One of Allie's closest friends, Ruth, came especially from Philadelphia to be with her. This never-ending fund of assistance helped us to know that we would be able to bring up our new daughter in an atmosphere of love and caring. The feelings of despair that sometimes seemed insurmountable were tempered by the knowledge that our friends were completely understanding of our situation. More importantly, they were completely accepting of Sarah.

2

WAVING, NOT DROWNING

If you come to a fork in the road, take it.

Yogi Berra

It was the middle of January. Sarah had been home for about ten days and needed an all-in-one outdoor outfit. I agreed to go and buy one and drove to the local shopping centre. This whole trip shouldn't take me more than 45 minutes – I was quite decisive about this sort of thing, and often bought the first item that caught my eye.

I parked in the multi-storey car park and wandered down to a big store which specialised in baby and toddler clothing. I stood looking at the rows of garments and considered the choices before me. What size would she need? Of course, there was no point in buying for a newborn baby, as she would grow out of it quite quickly. But then again, she's got Down's syndrome, and so she won't grow so fast. Now . . . what about the colour? Does it matter? Of course it does. I mustn't buy something garish which might draw particular attention to her – I wouldn't want that. But then I couldn't possibly choose a delicate shade because . . . well, she's unlikely to be petite or dainty. Pink was definitely out, because I didn't want anything 'girly', and I couldn't possibly buy anything in blue, as it would just be making an unnecessary political point for its own sake. Black was too funereal – I was already feeling depressed enough as it was – and white was virginal and impractical.

What about the expense? I couldn't buy anything too cheap, because then it might be assumed that I couldn't care less what Sarah wore and didn't value her enough. Then again, if I bought something too expensive, I would merely be over-compensating, which would be equally wrong. Oh, dear. This was getting difficult. No, it was no good, there was obviously nothing I could buy in this shop – I had better try elsewhere.

I went into another half a dozen outlets, but in each one the decision became harder and harder, and I became more and more confused. With every new shop, the level of anxiety grew. This was ridiculous – what could be more straightforward than buying some clothing for my daughter? But it was all becoming increasingly complicated, and turning into something much more significant than I'd anticipated.

In one shop I confided in a shop assistant, and rambled on for what seemed ages about the dilemma I found myself in. She was extremely nice and helpful, but I'm sure she hadn't the first idea what I was talking about. In another shop I became quite annoyed when the assistant was only able to show me one outfit: 'Just because she's got Down's syndrome doesn't mean I shouldn't have some choice for her!' The poor woman looked utterly bemused. I trudged out of the shop feeling absolutely desperate.

My shopping expedition finally came to an end when I stopped in my tracks in another shop: there, putting children's underwear out on the shelves, was a young woman with Down's syndrome. I stood and stared at her, not caring if she noticed me or other people saw what I was doing.

Waving, Not Drowning

Was this what Sarah was destined for? Would this be the most she might achieve as a job of work? Was this the most we could hope for? And yet . . . she might never be able to do even this kind of menial work – a job like this might well be beyond Sarah's capabilities when she grew up. What on earth did the future hold?

I hurried back to the car and drove the short distance home in floods of tears. Allie's mother Ursula happened to be visiting. I could hardly speak. 'I'm sorry, but I couldn't do it – I couldn't get her outfit. I'm sorry – I'm really sorry.'

Poor Ursula had never seen me so upset, and I felt very embarrassed that such a simple task had resulted in such an outpouring of emotion. Of course, we all knew that I wasn't just crying about a coat, and the reason for my tears was much more profound, but even at the time it did seem so pathetic. After half an hour of explanation, tea and sympathy, I decided – like the remedy for falling off a horse – I had to go out and try again. I went to another part of town and finally purchased this much sought-after garment. It would have been easier to find a Gucci original.

I had spent virtually the whole day searching for one piece of clothing for Sarah. Was this how life was going to continue? How on earth, I wondered, would we have time for any other family activity? Supposing we wanted to buy her a bicycle when she was older? I'd have to set aside a whole year. . . That particular day was one of the most depressing and upsetting of all since Sarah's birth. A supposedly simple act had manifested into a major traumatic event and symbolised all the ambivalent and ambiguous feelings I had about Sarah.

I was naturally still very bewildered, and soon realised that the only way I could manage was to try to return to the 'normal' routine: I was anxious to get back to work and try and pick up the pieces of ordinary life. I wasn't trying to avoid the situation – how could I possibly do that? Rather, it was a method of coping with the shock and the future ahead. I talked to my friends and family at great length, but I am by nature quite stoical and not a worrier. All right, so maybe I was reacting in a typically male way, but this was how it was. Unlike Allie, I didn't need to discuss every scenario endlessly: I just wanted to get on with things, and for these first, terrible few weeks to be over. Sarah's arrival had been a fluke: a case of what appeared to be poor fortune. But she was here now, and somehow we just had to manage.

It was ironic, because Allie and I had always considered ourselves lucky. We had both experienced happy, stable childhoods, and our families were healthy and financially comfortable. Up until the shock of Sarah's birth, we had led fairly charmed lives. Perhaps we had become too smug, too arrogant in our security, and this was how we were being repaid? Was it really bad luck or divine retribution? At the time it didn't seem to matter. I was too upset, too confused to think about it and soon . . . too busy.

Within the first month or two, there seemed to be a huge succession of helpers and callers, and the constant activity of visitors and telephone calls distracted us and helped us to survive. The immediate reactions of our families could not have been better. Allie's sister, Carey, was a great source of support – always happy to listen to Allie and offer sound and sensible advice. She undertook her sisterly duties with great sensitivity. She was faced with the added burden of adapting to her own role as an aunt of a child with Down's syndrome, and all the changing emotions and responsibilities that came with it. Being the older sister imbued her with a lifelong protectiveness which was cemented by this experience.

Waving, Not Drowning

I have read and heard of grandparents of babies with Down's syndrome whose preoccupation with their own outdated views and negative feelings has only created further pressures for an already struggling family. Our parents seemed to approach the situation with uniform acceptance. Doubt was never expressed about whether we would or should keep Sarah, and any secret fears were kept tightly under wraps. The focus for each of the four parents was simply to help us cope in any way that was required, and this was a tremendous relief to both of us.

Allie's mother's weekly visits became her most important emotional prop. Fortunately for me, Allie could empty herself of all her thoughts and feelings to her mother without feeling she was burdening her, which she often did sense she was doing with her close friends. That Ursula's feelings mirrored Allie's only enhanced this closeness. The mutual understanding was total.

Allie had to talk about all aspects of the situation from every possible angle – an unending stream of consciousness, worries, concerns, possibilities and likely and unlikely scenarios that had to be explored, dissected and then reassembled for further discussion. Every thought was expressed, no idea left unsaid. Desperate to find a reason for Sarah's existence, Allie was in turmoil. Key to it all was the moment of conception.

Sarah was conceived in Suffolk. Had we, Allie wondered, been too close to the Sizewell 'B' nuclear reactor, which blotted out the beautiful coastal landscape? She dwelt on all the circumstances relating to the moment of conception: had the quarrel she and I had had somehow tainted the atmosphere and destroyed any prospect of a happy outcome? If we hadn't argued, would there have been an earlier moment of conception, and ultimately a different baby? Allie obsessed about this and other possibilities *ad infinitum*!

A Major Adjustment

I understood that Allie was working her way through the grief by talking about Sarah constantly, but it was having the adverse effect on me. I had actually accepted Sarah for who she was amazingly quickly, and now needed to try and take stock of the situation and look to the immediate future, one day at a time. I felt I had to try and hold the family together, but Allie's need to talk all the time about 'what might have been' was making me feel more depressed.

Of course, Allie had to have the opportunity to talk about the situation as much as she wanted, and I didn't want to deny her this need. She had to visit friends, have people over, spend as much time and money on the telephone as she wanted. She had to attend as many self-help groups and meetings as she wanted – but I couldn't be involved at every turn. I also wanted to talk about the situation, but I just wasn't capable of devoting as much time and energy to all the whys and wherefores that Allie could.

The two of us had always operated very differently on an emotional level, but this was now a time of crisis, and we had to respect each other's coping mechanisms more seriously than ever before. I just couldn't handle this constant emotional barrage, and it was making me feel more miserable, frustrated and helpless. We had to strike up a pact. Allie had to channel her outpourings through other outlets.

It was amazing we ever made it out of the house in those first few weeks, what with all the talking that went on. Allie also found the thought of having Sarah observed and commented on very difficult. This was not made any easier by a remark made by a friend of Allie's, who had never met Sarah, and obviously felt it important to speak the unspeakable. During a telephone conversation he inquired, 'Do you feel like hiding her face when you go out?'

Waving, Not Drowning

Our first trip out as a family foursome was to the local shops to buy bunk beds for the children. Daniel was in a buggy, and I carried Sarah in a sling. We might have appeared the 'perfect' family, and indeed a woman actually remarked as much to us. This image seemed so far from the truth, and to belie the family's turmoil. We just wanted to retreat back to the privacy of our home and shut out everyone who didn't know the pain we were going through.

We were so distracted and disordered during this shopping trip that we ended up buying the first beds we saw – far too big for their room. For many years, the bunks protruded so far along the wall as to actually prevent anyone opening the bedroom door properly – a daily reminder of the confusion of those early days.

When we did take Sarah out in those first few weeks, we dreaded being stopped by people whose natural inclination was to bill and coo and ask all the usual questions about a newborn baby. People who didn't know us probably had no idea that Sarah had Down's syndrome, but we were absolutely convinced that it was on their minds and they just didn't want to say anything that might upset us.

Thus, complete strangers who happened to glance in Sarah's direction would be accosted and advised of Sarah's name, age and diagnosis – whether they were interested or not. Confession was the handshake. Passers-by, who thought they were merely passing by, were prevented from doing so with a ten-minute lecture on our situation. The faintest of smiles in our direction was the cue for an extended discussion on children with learning disabilities and all the attendant implications. No pedestrian was safe from Allie's watchful eye, should they show the slightest inclination to comment on our second-born.

However, after a while it dawned on us that people probably didn't even notice that Sarah looked different from other babies, and that even if they were aware of her having Down's syndrome, they were probably not interested enough to endure a long conversation. We were completely obsessed, and I'm afraid everyone we came into contact with at that time must have got really fed up with us.

The heart problem Sarah was diagnosed at birth meant needed a more detailed electro-cardiogram to ascertain its exact nature and seriousness, and she was referred to the Royal Brompton Hospital. Strangely enough, we weren't particularly nervous about this appointment, which was exactly two weeks after her birth. Life seemed to be so fraught with difficulty already that a potential operation or further medical treatment seemed almost insignificant against Sarah's future emotional needs.

I remember our appointment was delayed by about two hours, and we were finally led into the consulting room to be faced with a mountain of technological instruments and banks of electro-cardiogram machines. Naturally our hearts sank at the thought of our tiny Sarah being wired up to, and at the mercy of, all this technology. Amazingly, however, the consultant ignored all these appliances, preferring to diagnose Sarah's condition with just a stethoscope. He listened to the various rumblings and gurglings of her heart with the concentration and intensity of a man conducting an orchestra. His junior doctor, trembling with excitement at the thought of employing all the modern machinery at his disposal, seemed almost disappointed. Finally, the consultant reluctantly agreed to let his junior have his way and, with the relish of a young Dr Frankenstein, the medic hooked Sarah up!

Subsequently an ASD (Atrial Septal Defect) was confirmed,

meaning that Sarah had a hole in the wall separating the two atria of the heart. It was a common occurrence in children with Down's syndrome, it was explained, and should not have any permanent effect on her life or her life expectancy. With luck, the hole would close naturally in due course, and surgery would probably not be required.

Of course, in retrospect, if Sarah's heart condition had been serious, it would have caused us much more worry, and all our lives would have been further altered by this additional burden. The prospect of leading a 'normal' family life in the future would have been far more remote, as we would have been embroiled in a flurry of hospital appointments and procedures. Sarah's progress would have been further delayed, and there would have been even less time to devote to Daniel.

Nearly five years later, the same specialist in the same consulting room in the Brompton confirmed that the hole in Sarah's heart had actually closed by itself. We walked away from the hospital for the last time chatting happily about our forthcoming journey home, Allie and Sarah deciding what they were going to do that afternoon. Not only had we received the good news about Sarah's health but, in contrast to that first depressing appointment, we had also been reminded how different everything now felt.

There was another significant appointment during the first few weeks of Sarah's life: her existence had to be registered.

A friend of mine had worked temporarily in the Office of Registration of Births, Deaths and Marriages in south London. The Registry was run by a harridan of a woman, so completely insensitive and impervious to people's situations that her usual welcome when a member of the public approached the reception desk was barely to look up from her newspaper and bark, 'What are you here for? Birth, death or marriage?'

A Major Adjustment

This opening query didn't seem to change no matter what the state of the person on the other side of the desk. A woman dressed head-to-toe in black, sobbing uncontrollably, a nervously coy young couple, or a mother proudly clutching her newborn infant – all would be interrogated in the same bored, disinterested tone. Service with a sneer.

There was, however, very little humour to be derived from our trip to register Sarah's birth. So ambivalent were we about this task, normally one of pride and pleasure, that we had just not wanted to face it at all. It was not because we were unsure of a name. She was Sarah from the day she was born. It was also becoming easier to venture into the outside world. It was just that somehow this symbolic act of the baby becoming a 'real' person in society didn't seem appropriate – as though in our situation this act of registration would take on a separate process, with different rules and a different significance.

There was just one day left of the period during which the law required a birth to be registered when we finally took Sarah. We looked at the birth certificate sadly. Sarah Kate Merriman: a lovely name – but who was this Sarah Kate? If only we could peel away her Down's syndrome and behold the other Sarah Kate, our longed-for daughter. . .

By now we were beginning to have contact with a number of professionals, mainly from health departments. In addition to regular visits from the midwife, health visitor, GP and at least two physiotherapists, Allie also had to take Sarah for appointments with the speech therapist, hospital consultants and the community paediatrician. The comings and goings were constant, and Sarah seemed to be an endless focus of attention for all sorts of agencies and interested parties. It seemed we would never have enough time for ourselves or Daniel again.

Waving, Not Drowning

On Valentine's Day, when Sarah was five weeks old, Allie and I went to the Czech Club in north London to celebrate together. The Czech Club is a venue that John, Allie's late father, had frequented throughout his London life. It's a lively and yet peculiarly intimate club, originally for Czech nationals, in a house in a residential street. The restaurant is based in two rooms with a small number of tables, so I always feel I'm dining at a friend's house. This was the first time Allie and I had been out alone together since Sarah's birth. We wanted to have an evening away from the stresses and strains of our life, and I had naively hoped we could enjoy a relaxed evening together: a temporary if superficial respite from the constant drama.

It didn't turn out that way. Allie became preoccupied with the thought that Sarah would never have a Valentine's Day partner to celebrate with. She just couldn't allow herself to enjoy the evening, as she was convinced that a similar experience would always be denied her new daughter. If Sarah would always be deprived of evenings like this, how could Allie now allow herself this pleasure?

Allie was sad and quiet all evening, and when we got home she sobbed uncontrollably in my arms for nearly an hour. This was the first time she had let herself lose control so freely since Sarah's birth. She was crying for the 'fantasy' child that had disappeared, and for the dependent baby who had replaced it. This baby needed more love than most children, and yet Allie did not yet feel this love. Soon I was crying as well. We cried for the family we now were, and for the one we should have been. We cried for our daughter whose life would be so different to our own, and with whom we couldn't identify. We cried for the uncertainty of the future, and most of all we cried for the unfairness of it all. (I certainly did do a lot of crying at that time, but then I am so prone to emotional lability that I've actually been known to blub during *Pimp My Ride*.)

The need for parents to document the accomplishments of their children is a natural process. With Daniel, we would delight in his first words, exalt his first few steps and proudly display his early artwork. Virtually every week of his early life is documented on videofilm. By the arrival of the second child these events do not seem so remarkable, and usually there is not nearly so much detail kept. Of course this was not true of Sarah, because with her, every achievement was eagerly anticipated and marked. Her capabilities were a testament, not only to her determination to overcome her disabilities, but also to all the people who had helped us. Her achievements over the first two years enabled us to feel that we were doing as much as we possibly could for her, something every parent with a disabled child needs continual reassurance about.

During this period, we were always being asked if Sarah had learned to walk yet. It had become a major issue, and one that was beginning to worry us. Despite all the intervention, state-of-the-art baby walkers and much encouragement, she seemed to be getting nowhere fast. Actually, this isn't strictly true: she was getting somewhere fast, but by using her backside as a mode of transport.

We had become so tired of Sarah's bottom-shuffling. Because she had never crawled it was, at first, a relief to know that she could transport herself quite speedily on her backside, and then her somewhat idiosyncratic mode of movement was amusing. But by the age of two, we really felt she was ready to walk, and became extremely frustrated at her inability to do so. We began to wonder if she would ever feel the need to get up on her pins. She certainly didn't seem that bothered, but we were. . .

I couldn't wait for Sarah to be walking beside me, holding my hand. I didn't care how she achieved this, how ungainly or slow it might be: I just wanted to see her put one foot in front of the other! The matter of walking became powerfully symbolic: these first longed-for steps came to represent her first strides towards independence. If these could be achieved, we could then look with a new optimism at the road before us. Once she could walk, the contemplation of all other areas of delay would seem more manageable.

As a birthday present to her maternal grandfather, on 4 February 1994, Sarah finally walked unaided for the first time. It was still another two months before she could maintain any lasting motion and equilibrium, but the thrill of seeing her walk for the first time was breathtaking. The reward of each new stage is all the greater for all the investment involved. If Neil Armstrong thought he was taking a giant step for mankind with his first few steps on the Moon, he should have seen our reaction when Sarah completed what we considered to be the terrestrial equivalent.

Sarah was now beginning to do things for herself which showed that she had more than a basic understanding of the world around her. She watched how things were done and then copied them. She was gradually emerging from her chromosomal chrysalis into an individual with preferences, interests, and choices.

Looking back over these first two years, I find my over-riding memories are of the huge emphasis on stimulation, and the close scrutiny of each aspect of Sarah's development. That may appear a rather impersonal and unspontaneous recollection of a precious time with one's child, but it is not the whole story. Through these various activities, the everyday care of Sarah and the passage of time, a subtle but vital change had occurred in our feelings towards her. Sarah's diagnosis had become just one of the many facets of her being, and Sarah herself had come to life. She was now a little girl in her own right.

When Sarah was born, she was a Down's syndrome baby, who happened to be our daughter. Now, as time passed, she had become our daughter, Sarah, who had Down's syndrome.

3

IMBECILES, IDIOTS AND MORAL DEFECTIVES

Mongolian imbeciles are usually the offspring of feeble, immature or exhausted parents. Thus, an imbecile of this kind is often either the first child of young parents, the last child of a numerous family or the only child of elderly parents. Sometimes there is a clear history of maternal ill-health, debility or privation. Sometimes there is parental syphilis.

Francis Crookshank,
The Mongol In Our Midst (1925)

In the spring of 2017, scientists discovered the remains of a child in in Saint-Jean-des-Vignes, France, which, as far as we know, represents the earliest case of Down's syndrome in archaeological record. The skeleton of a young child, aged between five and seven, dated back to the 5–6th century AD, and the researchers found the skull had several features that were akin to Down's syndrome, including a short, broad skull and thin cranial bones. Furthermore, from the way that the child was buried, in the same manner as other skeletons discovered at the same time, prompted the researchers to believe that the child had not been judged differently, and may not have been stigmatised by the community for having the condition. Although by no means definitive, and open to speculation and debate, this find remains encouraging.

Down's syndrome has probably existed for about ten million years – as long as humankind – but history has mostly not been so kind to those with learning disabilities. According to Brian Stratford in his book *Down's Syndrome, Past, Present and Future*, the Athenians and Spartans deserted handicapped babies on hillsides to starve or be taken by wild animals. In Greek culture the handicapped were regarded not as human, but as 'monsters' belonging to a different species. In fifth-century Athens, 'democracy' only extended to the 'public' people – men, whilst slaves, women and the handicapped were not involved in civic matters and were therefore 'private' people. The Greek word for a private person is *idiotis*, and the word 'idiot' was still being used as a medical term of severely handicapped people as recently as the early 1970s. The word is obviously still in use, but only as a term of insult.

There is no doubt that the use of particular language and terminology throughout history has had a huge influence on the way people with Down's syndrome, and indeed other disabilities, have been treated. An inextricable link exists between legislation, words and social policy, and the attempt to use language that is less pejorative can only help in the understanding of disability. There is no doubt that any changes in words or idiom reflect the changes in our thinking.

As I wrote in *A Minor Adjustment*,

> the argument that language is not important is, I believe, misplaced, and the arrogant and condescending dismissal of certain words or terms as 'politically correct', and therefore supposedly a source

of amusement, is extremely annoying. Terminology is meaningful, and should not be dismissed as being trite and unimportant. It also does not mean that because time and energy is expended on this issue, other important battles of equality in education or employment are forgotten. It is the same battle.

Of course, one can always quote examples where the theory has gone too far, but that is not the point. 'Idiots', 'cretins', 'morons', 'imbeciles', 'half-wits' and 'fools' have all been used to describe children and people with learning difficulties. 'Mong' and 'spaz' are still used as terms of insult or abuse. I realise that 'learning difficulties' is not ideal, because I am well aware that Sarah's difficulties amount to much more than those of 'learning', but this, and 'learning disabled', are the terms by which adults in this situation wish to be described. Such terms are certainly more acceptable than 'mental defective' or 'retard', or even 'handicapped', with its connotation of street-corner begging and charity hand-outs.

I suppose there is the possibility of reclaiming the 'R' word (retard), which is still used as a term of abuse, particularly in the US. After all, African-Americans have managed it with the 'N' word. The gay community uses 'queer' as a positive description, and nowadays there is even 'Mad Pride', a movement that celebrates mental illness, and a 'BonkersFest', during which bananas are fired out of a cannon – both happily embraced by people with mental health problems. Not sure it would work with 'retard', though. I may set up a focus group. . .

Throughout history, thousands of children and adults with learning difficulties were needlessly imprisoned in institutions because they committed the crime of being different. Had she been born a generation or two before her birth in 1992, Sarah could well have been one of them.

Until the middle of the 19th century the treatment of imbeciles, congenital idiots, feeble-minded lunatics, dullards, mental deficients, moral defectives, mentally handicapped and subnormals, as the learning disabled have been referred to throughout history, had been one of distrust, fear and segregation. Workhouses, first established in the 1630s, were common in most market towns by the middle of the 18th century, and became the dumping grounds for 'the decrepit and dependent' of all descriptions. 'Institutionalising people', suggest Joanna Ryan and Frank Thomas in their book *The Politics of Mental Handicap*, 'is the way society deals with people it finds useless, dangerous or inconvenient'.

Then in 1845 the County Asylums Act compelled every county and borough in England and Wales to provide asylum treatment for all its 'pauper lunatics', and one of the first of these asylums was the Royal Earlswood Asylum in Redhill, a charitable institution which sought to aid the 'respectable poor' of Victorian Britain, which in 1852 became a hospital for 'idiots and imbeciles'.

It is possible that without a chance meeting in 1846, Dr John Langdon Down might not have become involved in what was to become a lifetime's work. According to a report in the *Medical Times,*

> Taking refuge from inclement weather in a country inn, John Langdon Down came across a girl – 'a semi-idiotic woman of feeble mind' – who was waiting on the party. Some years later, he described his feelings about her: 'A question haunted me – could nothing for her be done? I had then not entered on a medical

student's career, but ever and anon the remembrance
of that hapless girl presented itself to me and I longed
to do something for her kind.'

Langdon Down did actually do something for 'her kind'. He
was medical superintendent at the Royal Earlswood, and there
he extolled the virtues of separate institutional care and the
education of 'idiot children'. He emphasised the lack of scientific
education available to such children in 'pauper institutions', and
developed his own educational system for such children.

John Langdon Down was the first person to accurately
describe the syndrome which bears his name. Strongly influenced
by Darwin, he appeared to regard the retarded as evolutionary
throwbacks to inferior races. In 1866 he published a paper
entitled, 'Observations on an Ethnic Classification of Idiots', which
set out to classify the feeble- minded by arranging them within
various ethnic categories. At Earlswood he drew on written and
photographic material to distinguish a group of patients that he
described as 'Mongolian', because of the Mongoloid appearance
of their eyes. In this thesis he was, of course, both politically and
philosophically mistaken – and in any case, it was the epicanthic
folds on their eyes (the skin folds of the upper eyelid which
cover the inner corner of the eye) which constituted the primary
'characteristic' by which he was prompted to make his 'racial
type' identification.

By this time Langdon Down had come to realise that the need
for hospital places from wealthy clients was such that he could
profit as the proprietor of a private institution of his own. He
resigned from Earlswood, took up a Harley Street private practice
and set out a plan to open an institution for 'payment cases'. In
due course John Langdon Down was granted a licence to run

a private establishment at the White House, the property he purchased in Hampton Wick, just to the west of London, with his wife Mary.

The White House was renamed Normansfield in recognition of the Langdon Downs' solicitor Norman Wilkinson, and John Langdon Down assumed the title of Medical Superintendent. He and his wife developed the five acres attached to the house, and over the next 20 years acquired more properties and land, together with the river field running down to the Thames, until the whole estate comprised over 40 acres. In May 1868 the hospital opened as a private home for the 'care, education and treatment of those of good social position who present any degree of mental deficiency': Normansfield was to meet the need for a residential training and care centre for the learning disabled of the upper classes.

Initially, members of staff were recruited from the immediate vicinity, and several local families provided the mainstay of support. Langdon Down's intention was that the hospital should be run on the principles of a family home, its residents the members of an extended family. This was a somewhat pioneering notion for its time, but his rubric for the treatment of the institution's patients could fairly be described as revolutionary:

> The patient should be rescued from his solitary life and have the companionship of his peers. He should be surrounded by influences both of art and nature, calculated to make his life joyous, to arouse his observation, and to quicken his power of thought ... success can only be obtained by keeping the patient in the highest possible health. Diet should be liberal ... moral education is of paramount importance. He has

to learn obedience; that right-doing is productive of pleasure and that wrong-doing is followed by the deprivation thereof . . . he should be taught to dress and undress himself, to acquire habits of order and neatness, to use the spoon or knife and fork . . . the defective speech is best overcome by a well-arranged plan of tongue gym languages.

The Normansfield residents varied in age from toddlers to adults, and there were almost twice as many boys as girls. One of the institution's fundamental purposes was to educate patients in domestic and vocational skills and return them to their communities and families, by using as a system of rewards and punishments, but also some much more radical approaches. Through the creative use of role-play, particularly in 'shopping' lessons where pupils would act as shopkeepers or customers in order to learn the basic principles of money or weights and measures, John Langdon Down developed drama techniques that helped the residents become better integrated into society.

Staff were also trained in the use of sensory stimulation, and early forms of 'work experience' were even sought, in the hope that a few patients might be able to return to their family homes and lead some kind of independent life outside the institution. Developing educational opportunities for children with learning disabilities (a hundred years before it became government policy) and by using music and drama as therapeutic tools, Langdon Down treated each patient as an individual, whose unique potential, he felt, needed to be detected and nurtured. Despite Langdon Down's notions of racial stereotyping, his enlightened treatment of 'the idiots and imbeciles' and ground-breaking use of educational ideas, drama and music therapy is a unique story of dedication and vision. The hospital gained an international reputation for its treatment of the 'mentally handicapped' – a testament to the extraordinary foresight of the man.

The activities at Normansfield demonstrated Langdon Down's beliefs: teachers were engaged, and artisan workshops were developed at which young people could be instructed in crafts. Amongst other activities, there was riding, cycling, cricket, tennis and football. There were also Punch and Judy performances and donkey-cart rides, and every year over a hundred residents visited the Crystal Palace. The land was actively farmed, and a productive garden provided food for the kitchens and healthy physical work for the patients. Instruction was given in dancing, gymnastics, music and languages, and an elegant entertainment hall was built which was also used for Sunday services.

The entertainment hall, later known as the theatre, was open every Thursday evening, where there was the opportunity for any patient or staff member to sing, dance, recite or act, together or as solo performers. In order for the drama and music to be effective as a form of treatment, it was vital that the staff employed at Normansfield be not only skilled attendants, but also possess theatrical talent: the place was a sort of therapeutic Butlin's, whose staff, although not exactly 'Redcoats', were expected to be able to either play an instrument or sing.

John Langdon Down's work wasn't, however, purely philanthropic. Normansfield was entirely an institution for the learning disabled of the upper, genteel classes, who could afford private care for their relatives. Consequently, John Langdon Down and his family, supplemented by his Harley Street practice, made a vast fortune.

There were several reasons why such privileged families felt the need to have their children looked after in an institution. It wasn't that they couldn't provide physical care themselves: there was often a coterie of nannies, nurses and servants. In fact, many of these families sent their children away for positive reasons – they genuinely did believe that their loved one could be better cared for by experts, and certainly in most cases contact was maintained by visits and correspondence. Another motive for the hospitalisation of their children was to protect them: to arrange shelter from an outside world that could be extremely cruel. Some patients, however, were simply felt to be an embarrassment to their families, and needed to be kept a secret.

Although forever associated with the eponymous syndrome - the single most common cause of learning disability – John Langdon Down's work extended to other learning disabilities – he treated a number of patients on the autistic spectrum. Throughout his distinguished career, Langdon Down exhibited genuine concern, a pioneering approach and a true motivation to ameliorate the lives of the learning disabled. He was a long way ahead of his time, and was the first to recognise the potential of men women and children who had been discarded by everyone else.

John Langdon Down ran Normansfield until his death in 1896, and following his wife Mary's death four years later, their sons Reginald and Percival, who had both read medicine at Cambridge, took over the management of the hospital. The two brothers married, and both their wives played an active part in the running of the hospital. It is also somewhat ironic that John Langdon Down's first grandson, named in memory of his illustrious grandfather, actually had Down's syndrome and lived in the hospital until his death in 1971. Percival died in 1925, and the following year Normansfield became a limited company with Reginald at the helm.

The 1946 National Health Service Act, which came into force two years later, transferred local authority hospitals to the Ministry of Health. The NHS took over the major responsibility for mental health from county councils and boroughs, the main inheritance being a system of over 100 asylums, or 'mental hospitals', with an average population of over 1,000 patients in each.

By 1951, the Langdon Down family decided that it just wasn't practicable to continue to run Normansfield as private institution, and it was duly sold to the local hospital hoard. However, the Langdon Down family's involvement with Normansfield continued with the appointment as Medical Superintendent of yet another Langdon Down, Percival's son, Norman, who had been Deputy Medical Superintendent since 1946.

In 1961, Norman Langdon Down and 18 international experts in the disability field wrote to the medical journal the *Lancet* suggesting that the customary name for the condition, 'Mongolian Idiot', should be changed to 'Down's syndrome'. It took four years for this petition to have any impact, but in 1965, at the request of the People's Republic of Mongolia, the World Health Organisation agreed to this suggestion, and Down's syndrome subsequently became the globally accepted term.

Five years later, in 1970, Norman Langdon Down had stepped down as Medical Superintendent. His resignation brought to an end the family's involvement at Normansfield, a dynastic reign that had lasted just over a century.

The regime that succeeded his at Normansfield was not the NHS's finest hour, in some respects having the same gift for compassionate care as Basil Fawlty for hospitality. One patient at Normansfield during this time was Shelley Rix, the daughter of the actors Brian Rix and Elspet Gray. Shelley was born with Down's syndrome in 1951. Her parents were advised not to take the baby home, and Shelley was taken into a private home soon after her birth. 'That was the norm in those days if you had the resources,' wrote Rix in his first autobiography: 'the advice you received was to thank your lucky stars, put your mentally handicapped son or daughter in private care and get on with raising the normal members of your family.'

At the age of five, Shelley was admitted to Normansfield – a humiliating experience, in that the Rixes had to drag her through the bureaucratic processes demanded by the archaic 1913 mental deficiency legislation: Shelley had to prove that she was mentally handicapped, even though at that stage she could neither walk or talk. Brian Rix was even asked if he had venereal disease or was drunk at the time of conception.

The couple threw themselves into fund-raising events for the institution and Rix, then an actor-manager and known for his Whitehall farces, devoted his life to working on behalf of the learning disabled and became president of the learning disability charity Mencap. He was knighted in 1986, and six years later made a life peer.

I visited Brian and Elspet Rix ten years ago while researching my book, *Tales of Normansfield*. They were both delightful, and so welcoming, despite Shelley having only recently passed away. They clearly regretted the decision to have her institutionalised, and it was this that had motivated them both into their campaigning work. As I was leaving, Elspet drew me to one side and stage-whispered, 'Brian was so devoted to her. They had such a bond. I believe he sometimes thinks he gave birth to her himself.'

In 1988 a Green Paper was issued on 'Care in The Community', which suggested ways of moving money and care from the National Health Service to local councils and voluntary associations. Behind this recommendation was a strong endorsement of community-based care for as many current long-term hospital residents as possible: the report called for a determined programme of hospital closures, linked to a statutory duty and financial incentives for councils to make proper local provision.

Care in the Community applied especially to 'mentally handicapped', mentally ill and elderly patients. It suggested that 20,000 long-term patients (15,000 in mental handicap hospitals and 5,000 in mental illness hospitals) could be discharged 'immediately' if funds could be switched from the Health Service to local authorities. One positive was that, following the 1990 Community Care Act, the Department of Health officially adopted the less pejorative term 'people with learning difficulties'. Despite underfunding and bureaucratic difficulties, it did help some adults with Down's syndrome avoid the confines and indignities of institutionalisation.

In 1999 Normansfield itself officially closed, but through extraordinary serendipity, the Down's Syndrome Association now occupies office space in the former hospital buildings.

'Once you label me you negate me,' the 19th-century Danish philosopher and theologian Søren Kierkegaard declared, and it is true that every culture, creed or race is plagued by stereotypical views of its behaviour. Such identified 'traits' form the basis of discrimination, and the effects of ageism, racism and sexism are all still rife in society. People with mental illness and learning disability are no exception, and those with Down's syndrome are particularly prone to uniform, but uninformed opinion. They do, in fact, tend to be the subject of trite observations of a kind that would be considered abusive if attributed on a racial basis.

Adults or children with Down's syndrome are not necessarily either 'happy and affectionate' or 'stubborn and difficult to control'. There may be a number of people with Down's syndrome who are mainly happy and affectionate, and there may be a number who are also difficult and stubborn. Believe it or not, there may be some who are affectionate and stubborn! It may be true to say that some people with Down's syndrome are less socially inhibited, and that their emotions and frustrations are closer to the surface, but this does not imbue them with particular traits. There is in fact a great variety of characteristics and personalities within this particular community, and they possess a multi-dimensional range of emotions and attitudes.

But once people have become predisposed to recognise such stereotypes it is not easy to dispel them, and the public's perception of people with Down's syndrome will continue to be somewhat ill-informed and often patronising. We only see what we have been advised to look for. We tried to address some of the common stereo-typical views in one scene of *Minor Adjustment*. Amy, the little girl, has been admitted to hospital after a severe attack of croup. Her mother Sarah has stayed the night with her, and it is now the following morning.

Fade up: a hospital paediatric ward. Amy is playing in the background.

Woman: So, what's the matter with your child?

Sarah Oh, Amy's got croup. She only came in yesterday, but she's much better. I'm hoping we can go home today.

Woman: Yes. True. Has your daughter been in hospital before?

Sarah:	A couple of times.
Woman:	Oh dear. Poor thing. I suppose they're not very healthy.
Sarah:	*They?*
Woman:	Down's syndrome children.
Sarah:	Oh.
Woman:	I couldn't help but notice. Although she is very pretty.
Sarah:	For one of *them*, you mean.
Woman:	Oh, I'm sorry, I didn't mean to offend you.
Sarah:	It's all right.
Woman:	I hope you don't mind me asking, but did you know that she had Down's when you were pregnant?
Sarah:	No, I didn't.
Woman:	And you didn't have a test for it?
Sarah:	There was no reason to.
Woman:	Oh, I had all the tests with both my children. If anything had been wrong, I don't know what I would have done. I just couldn't possibly cope with a handicapped child.
Sarah:	Not everyone can. I'm certainly not saying every home should have one.
Woman:	Did you consider having her adopted?
Sarah:	No, not for a moment. Did you ever consider having your children adopted?
Woman:	No, of course not.
Sarah:	Then why do you ask me?
Woman:	Well, because . . . because she'll be dependent on you for the rest of your life.

Sarah: And your children won't be?

Woman: I just think it's a bit different. I mean, isn't it unlikely that your daughter will ever have a job ... or get married or ... have children of her own?

Sarah: And you're sure that both your children will have all those things. Aren't you lucky?

Woman: I suppose you've got some compensations. After all, they are meant to be very affectionate and happy children.

Sarah: Actually, Amy is both those things, but we like to think that's because she's Amy – not because she has Down's syndrome.

Woman: No . . . no, of course not. But there are certain traits, aren't there? I mean, aren't they supposed to love music and dancing?

Sarah: Yes. We're hoping she's going to be in the re-make of *South Pacific*.

Woman [*Pause*] Actually, in a way, my daughter also has special needs.

Sarah: Oh, really?

Woman: Oh, yes. Charlotte is extremely bright. She's been described as 'gifted'. Her school really don't stretch her sufficiently and we're having to get extra help. Of course, she is very advanced for her age.

Sarah: Why is she in hospital?

Woman: She fell out of a window and broke her leg.

Sarah: [*To herself*] So she's not that bright, then. [*Then, louder*] Well, I hope she's back on her feet again ... and back to school.

A Major Adjustment

Woman: Oh, that's all right. I've brought her in some work. I wouldn't want her to miss out.

Sarah: No, that would be terrible for you.

Woman: How old is Amy?

Sarah: Three . . . nearly four.

Woman: I know this might sound awful, but what sort of mental age is she likely to have when she's an adult?

Sarah: I beg your pardon?

Woman: Well, have the experts made any predictions about what she's going to achieve?

Sarah: No, they haven't, but she's doing very well – at her own pace.

Woman: I'm sure she'll make some contribution. I've heard of one who even worked in an old people's home. Everybody loved her.

Sarah: Amazing, isn't it?

Woman: Oh, there's Dr Thompson. I must have a word with her. You'll have to excuse me . . . [*Going off and calling*] Dr Thompson . . . could I just have. . .?

Sarah: . . . Stupid bloody woman. No wonder that girl fell out of a window – probably trying to run away from home. [*Sighs deeply*] Oh, I don't know . . . sometimes this is all too much. Come here, Amy. Mummy needs a hug.

Amy: Mummy. Mummy.

Sarah: [*Tearful*] Oh, Amy . . . I do love you. . .

Nurse: [*Approaching*] Are you OK, Mrs Stubbs?

Sarah: Yes . . . yes . . . thank you, Sister . . . I'm all right.

Nurse: You know, there's really no need to worry about Amy – she's much better.

Sarah: Oh, it's not Amy that I'm upset about. It's the people around her that worry me.

Fade down.

4

A MOTHER'S REFLECTIONS

Alison Wellemin

How does it happen that a situation so full of dread can transcend to one of deep contentment?

As I find myself contributing to this second book all these years later, and recollecting my anxiety during those early days over my daughter and our family's future, I now see a narrative of dwindling fear slowly being replaced by growing pride. As I got to know Sarah, she transformed from a bundle of my own anxieties into a vibrant individual with growing promise of a life fulfilled. The profound love I feel for Sarah nowadays arouses an intense excitement about her future quite unimaginable at her birth.

I wrote two chapters in *A Minor Adjustment*, and for the most part I am including them here in this new book, together with my subsequent reflections on the past 25 years. I want to launch right in with my original chapter covering the first two days of Sarah's life, where I told it as it was, with the bitter brutality that the experience held for me. I need to add that I was working at the time as a maternity social worker in the hospital where Sarah was born.

A Mother's Reflections

The hospital porter came to wheel Sarah and me to the post-natal ward. I wondered if he considered why I looked so glum after what is meant to have been such a glorious event. After all, there was this sweet, newborn baby, sleeping calmly beside me.

I knew my parents would be coming soon, and two thoughts struck me about how each would react. How on earth would my mother take the news? She had helped me take such tremendous care with every part of my pregnancy: ante-natal exercises (she used to be a physiotherapist), insisting on healthy eating and generally preventing me from doing too much whenever she could. Where had my mother's vigilance got us?

More superficial, perhaps, was the thought about my father. Would he bring his videocamera and record the early hours in hospital, as he had done with his other grandchildren?

I was wheeled into the side room of the post-natal ward and tried to avoid the looks of the other mothers who were milling around. I felt that I was in another world. The midwife helped me into bed and she left. I was alone with Sarah for the first time. I looked at her, peacefully sleeping, and felt nothing. No rush of love, of protectiveness or even pity. I picked her up mechanically and held her to try to evoke some emotion. I felt dead inside and returned Sarah to her cot.

My mother and father appeared and, soon after, Andy's mother (his dad was unwell and couldn't visit).

A Major Adjustment

Despite their obviously strained expressions, they were all loving and caring, and I began to talk about Sarah having Down's syndrome. They listened, without letting me know how they felt, preferring to let me talk. I, in turn, wasn't ready to hear their reactions.

My father had indeed brought his videocamera, and filmed the scene from time to time – at least this was no different from Daniel's birth. I loved him for this, as I did my mother for not even hinting at her own anxiety and pain.

Two young boys burst through the door – my nephews, Tom and Nicholas – to view their new baby cousin, and then my sister Carey appeared. I felt so envious of her: she had two 'normal' children and was never going to have to face the lifetime of hardship that I was sure was ahead of us. Carey was warm and welcoming of Sarah, whilst giving me space to make sense of what was happening.

What I only appreciated much later was how suddenly Sarah had changed everything for every family member. My parents were now grandparents of a Down's syndrome baby. Carey was an aunt of a Down's syndrome baby, and Tom and Nicholas were cousins of a Down's syndrome baby. New identities for everyone. The ripples were to go on and on.

Later, Andy returned with Daniel, who was wearing, I remember, his yellow Mickey Mouse sweatshirt. 'What have I done to you?' I whispered to myself as he came running in to see his new sister. I had planned not to be holding my second baby when Daniel visited, as all the books said this could help to reduce the levels of jealousy in the older sibling. That was one problem I didn't have. I wasn't holding her because I didn't feel like holding her. Photos were taken and we posed rigidly. For Daniel's sake I tried to look happy, but inside I was full of dread. Eventually the family departed, and Sarah and I were left to our own devices.

On the door of my side room was a sign which read: 'Do not disturb. Speak to a midwife before entering.' I was glad about this, as I was longing for some privacy and felt that I wanted to cocoon myself away for ever. However, this sign seemed to act not as a caveat but as an open invitation to all and sundry to drop in. I can honestly say that for the next couple of days my room was like Piccadilly Circus in the height of the tourist season!

The news of Sarah's birth spread like wildfire through the hospital, and well-meaning staff members from a multitude of disciplines all felt that they were ideally placed to pay me an unofficial visit. The hospital chaplain, the ante-natal sister, labour ward midwives, health advocates, interpreters, various con-sultants, an obstetric physiotherapist and a number of social work colleagues, as well as close friends and friends of friends –all popped in.

This furious activity served the function of keeping reality at bay. In retrospect, it seemed the more I talked to people, the more I could keep my mantle of control. I think what I was terrified of more than anything was the feeling of being pitied, or of Sarah being pitied. I was going to lead by example: I heard myself saying brave things about our lives becoming enriched, about the challenge ahead and about how I felt our family would become closer than ever.

When we were finally left alone again, I realised I was in overdrive, almost in a state of elation, and I certainly could not begin to sleep. Sarah was very undemanding. She fed well at my breast and dropped off to sleep. If only I could follow her lead. I was more drained and exhausted than I had ever been in my life, but sleep was to evade me for the whole period I spent in hospital and for much of the next month.

Soon after midnight, there was a knock at the door. It was the junior doctor who had been present in the labour ward when Sarah had first been examined. Although it was late, we talked for quite a while, and I was extremely impressed by her awareness, sensitivity and philosophical approach to what had happened. It seemed to consolidate some of the frantic machinations of the day's activities. She eventually took blood from Sarah, which would be sent away for likely confirmation of her diagnosis. Sarah screamed as the blood was drawn, and I was shocked to realise that I was so emotionally detached that I felt nothing about her cries of pain. I felt ashamed and guilty.

For the rest of the night I was in what seemed to be 'an icy grip' – a phrase I coined for the unwelcome feeling I was to experience intermittently for the next few weeks. I can only think of it as the palpable evidence of panic and the abject fear within me.

I continued my automated routine of feeding and changing Sarah when necessary, hardly wanting to look at the being who 24 hours before had kicked within me. In retrospect, I was lucky that Sarah was able to breastfeed so easily – something newborn babies with Down's syndrome sometimes have trouble with. If she hadn't, I don't honestly know how I would have been able to cope.

The following morning, a kitchen domestic bearing tea arrived and wished me a cheery good morning. She looked at the baby and asked if it was a boy or a girl. I told her it was a girl, and then felt a sudden need to tell her all about Sarah. I would have to face telling people sooner or later – why not now?

'Sarah has Down's syndrome,' I mumbled.

She let this sink in for a moment, looked at me and said, 'What have you been smoking?'

I tried to explain the facts, but there seemed no point as this accusation seemed so hurtful. I felt a complete failure, and looked away until she had left the room. She was soon followed by the cleaner, whom I also told about Sarah.

'Oh,' she said. 'You're a social worker here, aren't you?'

'Yes,' I said.

'Well, you've been listening to too many problems. This is what has made this happen.'

I could hardly believe what I was hearing, but realised that this was just the start of how we were now going to have to live our lives. Encountering ignorance, and prejudice – always being on the defensive and having to make explanations and excuses. I made a mental note that when I felt much stronger, I would like to mount a campaign to ensure that all hospital staff and ancillary workers were provided with some basic training and information about such situations. They were, after all, at 'the coal face', and would sometimes have to face people in crisis and turmoil.

The frantic visiting stopped after the second day and I had more time to reflect, and I thought of a close friend, currently in a room in an ante-natal ward, exactly two floors down from mine. She was also expecting her second child, and I remembered a recent outing with our sons, sharing with each other our secret hopes for a little girl this time.

Since then, there had been some complications in her pregnancy, resulting in her admission to hospital for several weeks. I had made a few visits to her side room, feeling fortunate but somewhat guilty that I wasn't in her position of being trapped and uncertain about the future. What would she be thinking now? I felt closely bonded to her, but sensed that it would be impossible to now pay her a visit. The depth of our joint fear and pain would overwhelm us both.

Soon after I had returned home, my friend told me that her little girl had only lived for four hours. We sobbed together, but were unable to console each other in our grief. At the time, although I naturally felt very sad for her, it seemed that I was worse off: not only had my child 'died' – I was, after all, grieving for the child that I didn't now have – but I also had a child that I didn't want. A child that needed looking after and caring for, and who might remain like a child for the rest of her life.

One of the midwives requested that I have lunch in the day room with some of the other mothers. I had to refuse, as I just couldn't face them. My feelings were so totally opposite to theirs of apparent joy. This was the first time I was to experience just how hard it was to be with other mothers and babies, and this was actually to last until Sarah was about four years old. Were we their worst nightmare? Did we fill them with dread? We would be a talking point: 'There but for the grace of God go I. . .' All the protocol around the arrival of a new baby was called into question. I longed desperately to stick to the game plan that I knew. I became very anxious to leave hospital. I had a vain hope that once Sarah was in our family's familiar environment, she would begin to feel like she belonged, that she was ours, and that my frozen heart would begin to melt. Surely, once she was in what was, after all, her own home, her rights would be established?

I felt tortured by my lack of love for this helpless creature who was so intimately mine. I had expunged Sarah's right to be loved purely on the basis of an extra chromosome.

As I read this chapter again, I realise how the emotions remain etched in my memory despite the fullness of time. I am struck, however, by how the raw ache has faded, and how much use I could have made of a crystal ball! I also have to confess I never did go back to train hospital workers who come into direct contact with patients, but strongly suspect the need for enlightenment persists.

A Major Adjustment

My second chapter in *A Minor Adjustment* covered the early days and months, and again I have kept most of the original text intact.

The most difficult time during those first few months following Sarah's birth was first thing in the morning. I would feel bleak and hopeless on waking and wondered how I would survive the day – let alone the rest of my life. I remember asking a psychotherapist friend of ours whether it was common when depressed to feel significantly worse when one first wakes up, and he responded wittily that I should read Freud's paper, 'Mourning and Melancholia'.

This intense deep sadness made me feel the urge to sleep in order to escape the real world. I remember having had the reverse feeling on finding myself awake after a nightmare, and being delighted at what was the reality. Now my reality had become a nightmare from which I wanted to flee, and my only method of achieving this was to sleep.

Fortunately Sarah slept through the night from day one. It was as if she knew that to exist within our family she would have to keep a low profile in those early weeks. I do wonder how I would have coped if I had been faced with the further exhaustion of broken nights during those weeks of turmoil.

The day's pattern seemed set. As the day wore on, life would take over and my spirits would lift. I clearly remember feeling almost jovial some evenings when friends and family gathered. At these times I would convince myself that my constant companion of dread was beginning to relinquish its grip . . . only for it to swallow me up again the following morning.

During the day my mind was in constant motion, my awareness heightened to such a degree as to be intolerable at times. My mind was in overdrive, everything seemed altered. Even ordinary familiar things – the view from our bedroom window – appeared different. Because of this, when I looked out I expected the players in the scene to perform in some other way. How could the man across the road still clean his car so obsessively and so regularly? Was he not aware that the world had changed so significantly and was now a different place for us? I loathed his lack of insight into our situation, which I would have thought would have given him different priorities. Of course, I soon realised that this was incredibly self-indulgent and arrogant. My life had changed for ever, but why should his? Who was he to know or care?

The love and care that was bestowed upon us during this period went a very long way in countering the feelings of despair. The phone became a drug at times. I needed a regular fix of support, and any opportunity to make sense of what was happening by way of some enlightening words that would ease my burden.

At the same time this telephonic dependence also became intrusive and exposing. I would be forced to explain again and again how we were managing. The words became repetitive, an empty, rehearsed mantra that only seemed to distance me from the caller.

We also made regular trips to the hospital where Sarah was born to see Dr Mackinnon, the consultant paediatrician. She was tremendously helpful, but I do remember thinking that although Dr Mackinnon was marvellous, she couldn't change the fact that Sarah had Down's syndrome. What really was the point of seeing her? What was the point of anything any more?

This question was answered in part when soon after Sarah's birth I met a young child with Down's syndrome. Jessica was then a year old, and the energetic grapevine had put us together. Her mother Bernice was a friend of a friend, and I had already been made aware of Jessica's existence at the time of her birth. I had even discussed with this mutual friend how I would never be able to cope if this happened to me, and how the prospect was so awful it didn't bear thinking about. Now here I was waiting to meet Bernice and Jessica and feeling fearful of how I would react to this little girl, who was a stranger but to whom my own daughter was so fundamentally linked.

I will never forget the broad smiles that greeted me as I opened the door. I almost forgot the purpose of their visit as the small child actively explored her surroundings, whilst her mother and I chatted animatedly. Jessica was inquisitive about the toys, about Sarah, and about everything around her.

Bernice was not the harassed and depressed person I had envisaged – quite the opposite. I was beginning to feel seeds of encouragement and hope as I talked to her and observed and played with her delightful child. My fears seemed to fall away.

Bernice did not deny her own shock and pain a year earlier, when her first, longed-for child was born.

However, experiencing them as they were now, and simply seeing that they had survived, was comfort indeed. Things that Bernice told me at that time have remained indelible in my mind.

The first was how at the beginning she had found it impossible to imagine waking up in the morning without 'Down's syndrome' rushing like a whirlwind into her consciousness. Now it seemed this was no longer the case. I remember feeling wholly doubtful that for me this process would pass as long as I would live.

The second vivid memory was of how Bernice spoke of her pregnancy: she had eaten healthily, refused alcohol and practised yoga. She was a midwife's dream! The irony was that something pretty drastic had occurred at the moment of conception that all her good efforts couldn't change.

I had done much the same thing, and had tried everything in my power to create a healthy environment for my unborn child. I had even taken things to the extreme, and made up rules such as not standing in front of the microwave oven. I realised I was being neurotic about it, and we joked about this. Andy said that instead of making sure I wasn't anywhere near the oven, I should actually climb inside the microwave so that the normal nine months pregnancy would only take four days!

I remember combining Bernice's and my joint experiences of our textbook approaches to the pregnancies and linking this to what I had read in a book about Down's syndrome by Mark Selikowitz.

'The presence of an additional chromosome adversely affects foetal survival: 80 percent of such pregnancies end in miscarriage. Children who are born with the syndrome may therefore be regarded as testimony to their mother's ability to support them during pregnancy despite this disadvantage.'

Could it be that the painstaking care we had both taken in our pregnancies had contributed to what could be considered as a far-from-healthy outcome?

I also remember a seminal telephone conversation with Bernice's husband Ian. I was bravely saying that at least we wouldn't have to worry about the evils of 'sex, drugs, rock and roll' as our daughters moved through adolescence. He quickly told me that he would not deny his daughter the prospect of experiencing these. He stopped me in my tracks. I had learned another new lesson. I began to look forward to future contact with this family. As a unit they had given me a massive boost to my level of adjustment and feeling of well-being. I needed to remain in touch.

The days passed, and I felt a sense of achievement for surviving another day, another week or another month. I had a strong instinct that if only time would pass quickly, everything would gradually feel easier. I wished time away and rejoiced as I turned another page of the calendar. I fantasised Sarah as an eight-year-old, and for some reason began to feel excited about this prospect. My future image of myself with Sarah was of a mother on an even keel coping and content with a daughter with a complete and beautiful persona.

A Mother's Reflections

Amongst the huge correspondence that we seemed to be receiving during this period were two letters that appeared to be circulars, and so were not opened with the usual enthusiasm until later in the day. I opened the first, and a leaflet featuring a photograph of a middle-aged woman with very obvious Down's syndrome features fell on my lap. The face looked up at me with childlike glee, and in very simple writing underneath this woman described the farm community she belonged to, stating that they required more funds. I was not prepared for this. I was not yet ready to contemplate Sarah's long-term future – after all, she had barely been born. I felt angry, and irrationally felt someone was attempting to torture me. I had been unfairly targeted.

I angrily opened the second letter . . . I had won first prize in the trade union lottery – a significant amount that I should have been grateful for at the time. Instead of being pleased at this good fortune, however, I felt unsettled, because I had never won anything in this way, and wondered why I had been singled out so mysteriously. The pleasure of winning money was superseded by a feeling of victimisation. Ordinary situations were taking on new rules and resonances, and I no longer felt in control of my responses to things.

I had lost all my points of reference.

My over-riding preoccupation was, why had this happened to me? At the time I thought that Sarah had Down's syndrome because I had wanted a girl too much, and this was somehow my punishment: I should have just accepted that the miracle of having a child was enough, and focused on my wish for a healthy one rather than on its gender.

However, I believe it did help that Sarah was a girl. I had my ideal family: an older boy and a younger girl. This ideal stemmed partly from my own childhood wish for an older brother, and was perhaps exacerbated by images in the media.

For some reason it was very important for me to dress Sarah in pink, or at least in girls' clothes. I had planned to put the second baby in Daniel's old clothes whatever its sex – partly for practical reasons, and partly because I had liked a tomboy image. I think what happened was that having had a label slapped on Sarah from birth, I didn't want her individuality compromised in any other way. There could also have been an element of desire to highlight the only aspect I felt proud of at that stage – that she was a girl. Irritatingly, this idyll of older boy, younger girl still persists. When I hear of a girl born after a first-born son I experience a pang of jealousy, which remains confused with the fact that I too have this pattern of offspring.

I began to think more philosophically about it, and I spent a lot of time desperately trying to discover a reason why this had happened to us. When there is no objective answer, I think the mind can search out and pinpoint almost anything. I decided that perhaps the circumstances that had caused us to conceive a child with Down's syndrome were predestined as part of a master plan, and that it was all beyond our control.

A Mother's Reflections

I had for a long time been aware that something would need to happen to me to jolt me out of my lucky and privileged existence. Alongside this, however, had been the contradictory feeling of 'It won't happen to me'.

I remember when Sarah was about two months old I was sitting with two of my dearest friends, who had both faced very difficult circumstances in their twenties. One had been seriously injured in a car crash, and the other had been stricken with cancer. Strangely, I understood that if I was to be tested, it would not be in the same ways as my friends. My challenge was to be the mother of a disabled child. This task would demand everything I thought I was good at. But what it now exposed to me was that I was not the warm, capable person I would have myself believe. I was a fraud.

I could not even love my own sweet baby daughter who was actually a joy to care for. She fed and slept well, and was soon to be smiling her beautiful smile. At other moments, rather than thinking I now knew the nature of the cross I was to bear, I felt that, as this unexpected thing had happened to me, so would everything else. The floodgates to potential disasters had been opened wide. I was no longer immune. I found it hard to face the outside world of babies and children, but for the benefit of all of us I knew I had to make the effort.

When Sarah was about three months old I eventually dragged myself to a mother-and-toddler group. This particular group, unsurprisingly, seemed to be totally centred on pregnancy, birth, babies and pre-school children. Discussions seemed to involve very little else. I suspected Sarah and I were objects of morbid interest. We were their worst nightmare – objects of pity.

This was perhaps purely my own perception, born out of intense envy of other mothers whose children were 'perfect'. I resented what seemed to be mindless moans about feeding difficulties, sleeping problems, feelings of isolation – all the things I had enjoyed talking about following Daniel's birth. At that time, comparing notes on baby minutiae had been my major preoccupation. I remember one woman at this group whingeing about what seemed to me a most insignificant setback in her birth plan. I had to bite back the words I wanted to say: 'Well, you had your perfect daughter at the end of it, so just be grateful for that!'

I did find this playgroup experience very difficult at the beginning. It highlighted the differences in our situations, and illuminated my vulnerabilities and dark side. However, after some weeks I actually started to relax and even enjoy myself. Once we had gone beyond obsessing about baby care, I realised there were some very stimulating women in the group, with a multitude of interests and backgrounds. I was reminded of other worlds and existences, and through this I rediscovered myself. I had taken such a confidence-knock as a mother that I had lost sight of my abilities. Through my involvement with some of these people I felt affirmed.

A Mother's Reflections

As well as this unexpected outcome for myself, Daniel needed to be given every chance to mix with friends of his own age. I like to believe my parenting of Daniel did not suffer to any great degree at this time of turmoil. On many occasions he lifted my gloom and I appreciated him more than ever.

It must have been very hard for Daniel in those early weeks. I would sometimes be unable to stop myself crying in front of him. I was aware of how children believe the reactions of their parents come about because of something they themselves have done, or who they are. I was very keen to dispel any feelings of this kind, should they have existed. I explained that my feeling sad was nothing at all to do with him, and that I was sad because it would take Sarah longer than other children to learn things. I told Daniel that Sarah had Down's syndrome, as I wanted these words to feel familiar. Words that could be expressed honestly and even perhaps one day . . . proudly.

My feelings for Sarah during those first few months very slowly began to change. Mere duty turned into feelings of protectiveness, which in turn reflected flickerings of wary love. However, I remained almost continually aware of her diagnosis. I felt ashamed that any loving feelings were still so tentative, inconsistent and dispersed. I had always imagined that whoever my child was, whatever and whoever they would become, I would love them unconditionally. This was not now the case. There was a condition. Normality. This was my requirement, and I hated my deluded self. Sarah was healthy and objectively a delight to mother. Sarah made perfect sense. It was me. I was the one who couldn't make sense of Sarah.

As I reflect on my anguished self, I know my thoughts sound shameful. I now realise how my response was a universal one when facing such a situation. Mercifully, I have grown to fully understand my reaction as part of a grieving process, nowadays accepted as an implicit part of the human condition where loss of any kind is experienced. Sarah now makes perfect sense to me, but it took a long time to adjust my expectations and see her for who she is. We started from scratch in those dark, early days, and by so doing slowly began to focus on and take pleasure in each tiny progression or sign of delight.

Regrettably, societal norms still mirror my early feelings towards my daughter. I am aware of the chilling fact that, despite loving my children equally (albeit in differing ways), at a certain stage of their gestation society would have authorised, even encouraged, the obliteration of one of them. Twenty-five years later this distressing fact is more pertinent than ever, as science evolves and moves towards seeking to eradicate potentially joyous and wholly fulfilled lives.

I am aware of how whimsical it sounds, but nowadays I honestly feel blessed that I am a mother of a person with Down's syndrome. I think this sense of good fortune has only arisen since Sarah's permanent living situation has been finalised: with the weight of responsibility lifted, I can simply enjoy Sarah for who she is and the life she leads. Contradictions persist, however, as this lucky feeling is challenged when I hear of an imminent birth, and know each time I am willing the baby to be 'perfect'.

My sense of visceral connection to and affection for babies and individuals with Down's, including those I have never before met, continues to surprise me. I first became aware of this when Sarah was in secondary school and we spoke at a Down's Syndrome Association conference in Blackpool for new families. At this point, the thrall of babies had been long lost on me, but here, greeted with a full crèche made up solely of babies and toddlers with Down's Syndrome, I found myself enraptured.

The support groups we ourselves attended along the way, including one still running in Norwood, the charity where I now work, have been a lifeline, mainly due to the power of a shared identification. Many families have become close friends, and their presence sustains me to this day. In earlier times, I would describe such groups as my refuge, the only place I could go where I would feel like other parents. We were not going to be singled out as different, we weren't on show, we didn't need to explain to each other why we were there – the mutual understanding was palpable and sustaining.

Various TV and newspaper interviews took place when Sarah was a child, and I confess I was not very skilled at such undertakings. In a live television interview with the lovely Caron Keating she asked me what the hardest thing was about having a child with Down's Syndrome. I blurted, 'She's Sarah and we love her,' and for some reason kept repeating this mantra over and over like a stuck record. Thankfully, I was rescued by Andy who, with far more experience of being in the spotlight, eloquently recounted our worries about the future, especially when Sarah reached adulthood. I soon realised I would never have the skills for public speaking and media interviews, only later to discover that Sarah had inherited this expertise from Andy.

I know it is impossibly hard to know what to say to a parent who has recently given birth to a disabled child, and I am loath to imagine how unprepared I must have been in the past to address such a situation. However, in my own experience it tended to be the ordinary 'wo/man on the Clapham omnibus' who got it just right, with comments such as 'She will be made of strong stuff,' leaving me feeling hopeful and positive. On the other hand, encounters with some of our therapeutically trained acquaintances saw clumsy or insensitive comments delivered with furrowed brows. 'Don't you just want to cover her face with a blanket when you take her out in the pram?' *No, actually!* And, 'She will remain vulnerable as she gets older – you probably worry about the risk of sexual abuse in the future.' *My child is not yet a year old, I am already fraught with anxiety, I hadn't actually thought about that one yet, but thank you, I have just added it to my list!*

It has been clear to me that some professionals in the field could benefit from greater awareness and insight. When Sarah was eight I attended a talk for parents of children with Down's by an 'expert' from the renowned *Tavistock Institute* of *Human Relations*, alongside families with babies and children of all ages. It turned out to be an unnecessarily negative presentation, during which the speaker proceeded to make a range of assumptions, including how we must never make the mistake of believing a person with Down's Syndrome will ever really enjoy their birthday, given that their arrival into the world will forever be linked to sadness. If only that speaker could see the thrill that Sarah and her friends take from these occasions, blissfully planning and celebrating each year's event, milking every moment to the last.

In an article in the *Independent* in 2005, I described how I was worried that life was going to be much tougher for Sarah, noting that friendships were becoming more difficult to make at her mainstream school. 'She is often on her own,' I wrote. 'She seems not to mind, but it breaks my heart.' What was occurring, I now realise, was that the gap between herself and her peers was widening. At the same time, her relationships with other children with Down's syndrome were becoming increasingly important as her sense of identity became more significant. She was beginning to understand difference, and attach meaning to the words of her diagnosis. At this stage she would list some of the physcal characteristics, but would then enjoy listing all her friends who shared her identity, thereby beginning to make sense of their differences.

While I was pregnant I had longed for a 'chip off the old block', hoping for a daughter in my own image. Initially, therefore, I struggled to accept Sarah's physical features, as they appeared to relate to an identity entirely different from my own. I had a lot to learn, of course, and was also yet to discover how difference can be a blessing – what I wouldn't have given as a teenager in the early seventies for a cute nose and long, silky, straight hair!

Sarah's influence has not just enhanced my personal life but has also been of enduring benefit in my professional sphere, as a social worker of 36 years and counting. My roles include various jobs with children and families within local authorities, a charity, in the NHS (CAMHS) and as an Adoption Panel Chair. Being a mother of a disabled child in these positions has opened up an understanding that extends across a breadth of realities, and hopefully has held me in good stead in my work.

Sarah has touched the lives of many. I am in awe as I watch others around her in matched admiration: Sarah speaking at major conferences; Sarah and her boyfriend Leon serving us Sunday lunch on the deck of his flat; Sarah answering many more pub quiz questions than me with her expertise in music/film/TV; dancing with unrivalled style and grace at her cousin's recent wedding; her sharp intuition which never fails to astound me – and so the list goes on.

A Major Adjustment

Another source of wonder is Sarah's integrity, and ability to confront others where others fail or fear to do so, in a sensitive, natural way that compels people to listen or instantly change their behaviour. She possesses an uncanny knack of putting people off their guard. I remember how Sarah once challenged my father when he raised his voice unnecessarily, and by doing so stopped him in his tracks, his face dissolving in a remorseful smile. Or I think of our dear friend, Annie, Sarah's godmother. Everyone else had given up trying to stop her smoking, but Sarah was unprepared to let it go, and kept up her caring refrain, over the years, until Annie's last breath.

Sarah's stance on life as a child and adolescent was naturally to focus on what was happening here and now, free from worries ahead. It taught me to live more in the present, and I still try to follow her lead. In recent years, and probably due to her maturity, Sarah now tends to ruminate more on future concerns, and I'm left wondering where wisdom truly rests in relation to our definition of intelligence.

My musing on being Sarah's mother is of course boundless. I will seek to close my reflections by conveying the profound pleasure our relationship has brought. A recent Mother's Day card she sent suggests that the feeling is mutual.

HAPPY MOTHERS DAY.

You're the greatest Mum in the world I love talking with you and deep down you understand what im feeling I love you so much I miss our past Together me and you I love you loads Best Mum 4 EVER.

5

THREE'S COMPANY

Dear Mary: We all knew you had it in you.

Dorothy Parker,
telegram to a friend who had given birth

Immediately after Sarah's birth Allie had raised the question of having another child. Here is what she wrote in *A Minor Adjustment*.

> Within an hour of Sarah's diagnosis, I was jolted by a conflict so powerful that it was to take a relentless hold on me. My first thought was that I would just have to have another baby. Somehow this would make everything all right again. I must have managed to gain a shred of rationality, however, for my next thought was that there must never be more children. My mission in life was to help and provide for Sarah – further offspring could only diminish this aim.
>
> Before I knew it, I realised that it wasn't a question of choice. It wasn't to be a conscious decision. The need for another child was overwhelming. It was almost beyond my control, and was to consume all my waking hours.

A Major Adjustment

We had planned to have just two children. If all had gone as expected and Sarah hadn't had Down's syndrome, I believe we would not have seriously considered having a third child. But here I was becoming obsessed with a third child even before I had left the labour ward with my second one!

Andy was very clear that my wish for another baby stemmed from the fact that I hadn't accepted Sarah and wanted to replace her. I thus felt trapped in the most dreadful bind. I would somehow have to learn to love Sarah, who at that time felt little more than a physical and emotional burden. She had taken the place of another – the one I had really wanted.

The desperation I felt at this stage could also have been due to my intense feelings of helplessness. I did soon realise that the birth of a third child would not make any of the difficulties associated with Down's syndrome go away, but I felt strongly that it would at least help in some way. I had to do whatever I could to rid myself of this sense of powerlessness.

At this stage I felt I just couldn't begin to contemplate another huge decision so soon after such a traumatic event, and I refused to discuss the matter, hoping that in time Allie wouldn't feel so desperate. I felt we would need to devote much more time to Sarah than to a non-disabled child, and I just didn't have the energy to give to another possible addition to the family. There was Daniel to consider, and I was already aware that his needs had occasionally been overlooked in all the attention Sarah had received.

Allie again:

Andy and I had never had differences before when it came to major decisions in our lives, and here we had no middle way. As time went by, Andy's original fear of Sarah being marginalised was no longer of relevance. He now knew that my love for Sarah was total, and the issues for me were in no way connected to any feelings of replacing her.

I needed my last experience of pregnancy and childbirth to be as totally joyous as my first time had been – how it was meant to be. My whole identity as a woman and mother had been affected to the core. I knew that I could never feel comfortable again hearing of another woman's pregnancy or news of a newborn baby. I was so sure that by having another experience (and I couldn't let myself consider anything going 'wrong') a healing process would take place. I too could again enjoy the luxury of 'the perfect experience' and lay to rest my bitterness.

Also of great importance was the feeling of 'invest-ment' we perhaps mistakenly make in our children. With two non-disabled children we could keep our expectations completely open. For Sarah, our aspira-tions had become very high, but nevertheless remained within certain limits. I no longer felt I had problems with this as it related to Sarah, but for our family as a whole I needed to be able to enjoy the privilege of all the hopes and dreams that parents of two 'ordinary' children can afford. After all, there had to be the pros-pect of the doctor *and* the lawyer!

There were other reasons too. If we did have another child then perhaps Daniel could share any responsibilities as well as other pressures that may be present in being the only non-disabled child. Also, for Sarah, I felt it would be healthy if she was not the 'baby' in the family, and that she would enjoy and benefit from a younger child growing up behind her. With three children, there wouldn't be the 'normal one' and the 'disabled one'. We would just be a family with all sorts of different children.

In the light of all this I felt there was an urgency to get on with the process. We weren't getting any younger, and the gap between the new child and Daniel and Sarah was increasing. We were in the swing of having young children. We were used to sleepless nights, being surrounded by nappies and toys. We didn't know how long it might take to conceive, and I felt all the risks in pregnancy were gradually increasing.

After a couple of months of fruitless 'negotiation' we agreed that we would not talk about another baby for a year – until Sarah's first birthday. Then regular discussions and negotiations took place with the preparation and tension of a UN summit. There was a great deal of strain on our relationship – we were just about coping with Sarah's existence, but now the far-reaching consequences of her birth seemed to be taking more of a toll on us. Allie again:

> The critical fact remained. Andy did not want a third child. I did. I was convinced that a desperation *for* something had to outweigh a desperation *not to have* something. I realise now that this belief was flawed and this was born solely out of the very

yearning I felt. The only time that I felt able to listen to Andy's point of view was when he talked of how our relationship could suffer as a result of having another child when our feelings in the matter were so opposed. I felt, however, that our relationship could equally suffer if we didn't have another baby. My most crucial concern was that Andy would end up resenting the child, although when I asked him about this he told me he was much more likely to resent me. I realised that this was not exactly the ideal way to bring a new child into the world, but I felt that I could cope with this dichotomy. I also believed that our relationship was strong enough to survive the impact of any resentment that would come my way.

I know Andy felt that this acceptance of the risk to our marriage was an insult. He felt that I didn't value our relationship enough, and that a third child meant more to me than having him, Daniel and Sarah. If they all meant as much to me as I said, why would I not be satisfied with our existing family?

I had great difficulty explaining how the issues were quite separate. My need to complete our family in this way had no bearing on what I actually felt for each of them. It would be fair to say I became quite obsessed with the prospect of a third child. When I looked at Daniel and Sarah I often imagined another smaller version beside them. I occasionally dared to fantasise a name which went well with 'Daniel' and 'Sarah'. I used to tell Andy of every couple who had increased their family beyond two children – definitely the current fashion. I felt my life was on hold until this decision was made.

People said to me how brave I was to contemplate having another child. I was sure, however, that I would have needed a greater amount of courage to consider living without a third child and deny what was an irresistible urge. Never believe that the desire for a subsequent child can't be as strong as it is for a first child.

I couldn't agree to a new baby, and yet I couldn't bring myself to say that we could never have another child. Doubts began to appear. Maybe it would be a good idea for Sarah to have a younger sibling to play with? Perhaps it would be fairer to Daniel to have some sibling support? Allie, meanwhile, was becoming more and more unhappy. I knew that if we didn't make a definite decision soon we would be in real trouble.

Towards the end of Sarah's third year I decided that Allie was not going to change her mind. If I didn't agree, she would be resentful towards me for the rest of her life. She would never forgive me. Maybe it would be for the best. I just didn't know.

Allie:

> After much soul-searching, Andy accepted that a third child was inevitable.
>
> At the end of June 1995 a pregnancy test confirmed my hopes and, although I was obviously delighted, the sobering realities of what lay ahead tinged my excitement. This pregnancy was going to be endured, not enjoyed – that experience had been lost for ever.

Three's Company

But with our third pregnancy Allie and I were now faced with a difficult dilemma. Following Sarah's birth, we were obviously much more aware of what could 'go wrong'. Our love for Sarah couldn't have been deeper, and we wouldn't change her in any way, but the thought of having *another* child with a disability was terrifying. We just didn't see how we could cope with another youngster with Down's syndrome, and part of the reason for having a third child was to provide some support and security for Daniel and Sarah. Sarah might need our help for the rest of her life – how could we provide a lifetime's commitment of this kind to two children? And how on earth would it affect Daniel? The chance of us having another baby with Down's syndrome was considered to be about one in a hundred, but we decided that we couldn't possibly go through the pregnancy and not know what the future held. As Allie wrote at the time,

> I could not bring myself to truly get in touch with what we would do if I found I was carrying a second child with Down's syndrome. To have a termination in ignorance of the facts must be traumatic enough, but to have an abortion in the light of the fact that we were obliterating an existence because it was like the daughter we have and love deeply would be impossible. A betrayal of Sarah and all those with Down's syndrome.

We decided to have a diagnostic test, in the hope of gaining the reassurance we needed, desperately hoping that an impossible choice would not have to be considered should we find we were expecting another child with Down's syndrome or any other disability.

A Major Adjustment

Joel was born on 1 March 1996, and my over-riding emotion was one of pure relief: relief that he was well and healthy and didn't appear to have any obvious disabilities – which was, after all, one of the main reasons for having an additional child – but a relief also that we didn't have to talk about the subject any more! Of course, looking back, I know that having him was the right thing to do. Our family wouldn't be complete without him.

We wondered whether Sarah in particular would find it very difficult to cope with a new sibling who would demand much of our time and energy. From the moment she had arrived, she had been the recipient of much attention, and we were sure she wouldn't take kindly to being out of the limelight on occasions. She overheard us telling a friend that her nose would probably be put out of joint, and she soon picked up the idea, saying, 'New baby. . . My nose out the window.'

In fact we were quite wrong, and Sarah wasn't adversely affected at all. She took to Joel straight away and adored him. Sarah was never jealous of him, loved his company and used to state repeatedly, 'I love my baby brother,' before adding politely, 'and my big brother.'

6

RING, RING GOES THE BELL

Come and put my brain in please Mr. Head
Sarah Merriman, aged eight

An Italian grandmother is walking on the beach with her grandson.

Suddenly a freak wave comes in and sweeps the little boy out to sea. Distraught, and not knowing what to do, the grandmother looks to the heavens. With tears streaming, she calls out, 'Why, God? Why? Why did you take away my beautiful grandson, who had his whole life in front of him? I know I could have been more devout, but I've always believed in you. I promise I'll go to mass every day if you can perform a miracle. Please bring my grandson back.'

Almost immediately, another huge wave crashes to the shore and deposits the grandson safely on the beach. His grandmother hugs him, checks he is unhurt, then looks to the sky again and calls out, 'He had a hat.'

Nothing is quite enough when it comes to our kids. We want everything for them, and our anxieties are endless. Parents are forever in a state of self-doubt over how they are performing, and whether they are really doing the very best for their children. The health and happiness of the children is paramount. When you have a child with Down's syndrome, you experience all the ordinary concerns, but with the extra worry that your child is even more vulnerable than most. It is your responsibility to safeguard without over-protecting. As I wrote in *A Minor Adjustment*,

> Knowing within an hour of her birth that Sarah had a disability certainly made it much more difficult to feel immediate love for her, but at least on a practical level we knew – from an extremely early stage of her existence – that she was going to need a lot more help than Daniel. Everything from feeding to toilet training, from talking to walking, was going to take longer with Sarah, and we would have to be patient. It's strange that, looking back, there wasn't one professional during the first year that would commit herself to the fact that Sarah would walk or talk.
>
> In Down's syndrome developmental delays are evident from the early months of life, in terms of children's ability to turn over, sit, stand and walk. The delay in speech and language is even more marked, the reasons for which are still not fully understood. We were advised, however, that there were three vital things that Sarah must have in her first year. Stimulation, stimulation and stimulation. Thus no stone was left unturned in efforts to produce a response from Sarah.
>
> Mobiles (we had more than a trailer park) were hung from every possible place, toys were poked and rattled in Sarah's face with monotonous regularity, and we constantly engaged in babbling and gurgling, pulling faces, singing songs, clicking fingers and clapping hands. We gave her objects to bang together,

different textures to touch and feel, we stroked her fingers to help improve manipulation, we massaged her to help tone up the muscles. Poor Sarah was probably desperate for some peace and quiet, but by God she wasn't going to get it when we were around. No possible motivational moment could be lost. This girl's full potential would not be left to chance. She must be stimulated to within an inch of her life!

The future goal was independence, in whatever shape or form and in whatever context Sarah could cope with, but to achieve that independence Sarah had to be dependent on lots of people. With years of education before her, Sarah would need extra support in playgroups, nursery and school. And this would not be an easy path, as until 1971 children with Down's syndrome hadn't even been given the right to any education, and only some ten years later were allowed attendance within 'inclusive education' in mainstream schools.

As Sarah Boston wrote in *Too Deep for Tears*, 'For almost all parents, the way forward to wider social acceptance of their child is through education. Only this kind of contact, they feel, can break down the barriers of ignorance and fear.' It is probably for this reason that the education of children with special needs is an issue that causes more dissatisfaction, frustration and argument than almost anything else.

In England and Wales, categories of pupils requiring special educational treatment were first defined in 1959 in the Handicapped Pupils and Special Schools Regulations. Twelve years later, the law was altered to establish a new category of schools which brought all children – regardless of the degree of handicap – under the care and jurisdiction of Ministry of Education. No child could be deemed ineducable. The responsibility of educating children with learning difficulties transferred from the Department of Health to the Department of Education – a symbolically important move. A Royal Commission emphasised the need to integrate as many children as possible into mainstream schools, and the Education Act of 1981 stated that a child has 'special needs' if he or she has a 'learning difficulty', and provided a number of important safeguards for the child, the parents and local education authorities.

The main change brought about by the Children and Families Act of 2014 in terms of learning disability is the replacement of the Special Educational Needs 'statement' by an Education, Health and Care Plan (EHCP) to support students, but in practical terms the actual effects aren't that different. The commissioning and planning of services for children, young people and families will be run jointly by health services and local authorities, and the EHCP extends the rights to a personal budget for the support needed by children, young people and families. Local services available to children and families must be made available in a clear, easy-to-read manner – this is usually called the 'Local Offer' – and, in addition, local authorities must involve families and children in discussions and decisions relating to their care and education, and provide impartial advice, support and mediation services.

There are some issues with EHCPs, such as difficulties in people understanding how they work, getting the necessary reports/ evidence and provision to match (as was the case with statements), and agreeing and writing into them desired outcomes. There is also concern about whether local authorities will have transferred children and young people over to EHCPs by the deadline of April 2018, and that rushing them may result in poor plans.

In addition, since the mid-1970s local authorities have been cutting back on spending, and more financial constraints under the respectable-sounding euphemism of 'Austerity' have prevented many councils from discharging their responsibilities. The situation for local authorities deteriorates with each passing year. A postcode lottery still exists on resources, and cuts to Legal Aid have hindered parents in taking their local authorities to tribunal in order to get the support they need. Pupils with special educational needs are being 'pushed out of sight and out of mind', according to the Ofsted chief inspector Amanda Spielman, who also criticised headteachers who exclude pupils they fear may drag down results, to improve their schools' position in league tables.

Sarah's own education started at age three at Hilltop playgroup which Daniel had attended two years previously. In the meantime, Daniel had started to attend Bounds Green School and, following the statementing process, Sarah followed suit two years later. The nursery class staff treated Sarah's arrival with ebullience and expertise. Her progress was monitored by regular reviews, planning meetings attended by teachers, speech therapists, a special educational needs co-ordinating officer (SENCO) and input from an educational psychologist.

We were made aware that people with Down's syndrome have a more developed visual perception than auditory perception. To complement the spoken word, the use of signs can ameliorate communication at an early stage. The Makaton method of 'signing' was introduced to us as the best method to help Sarah develop her speech and communication skills. The staff and pupils took to the Makaton sign language with great gusto. Within a few months the pupils had learned a few basic signs, and a special Makaton assembly had been presented to the rest of the school. I would arrive in the morning with Sarah to be greeted by various toddlers using the Makaton for 'Good morning'. So often did all the children use this sign – a thumbs-up followed by moving the hand across the chest – to greet the staff as well as each other that one teacher remarked she spent so much time using it she felt 'like a priest!'

Sarah settled in at infant school as easily as she had done in the nursery. Every morning the register would be taken and, with an intake of pupils from a wide variety of cultural and ethnic backgrounds, the children were encouraged – rather than just saying 'Here' – to state their presence with a salutation in any language they choose. Daniel, who was very proud of the fact that his maternal grandfather was born in Prague, had decided to adopt the Czech greeting of '*Dobry den*' (Good day). One morning, a fortnight after Sarah had started at infant school, Allie decided to see how Sarah would respond to this. She hid in the corridor whilst the register was taken and waited for the name of 'Sarah Merriman'. Would Sarah realise what this was about? Would she be aware enough to reply? Would she do so quickly enough, and if so, how would she cope with her limited language?

As her name was read out, Sarah, with great concentration and perfect accent, responded with . . . '*Dobry Den!*' Of course, she was only copying her brother, but it was very gratifying to know that Sarah – a child with special educational needs – was well on her way to being bilingual in English and Czech!

Every step of the way was encouraged by the school staff, and each of Sarah's achievements was greeted with great enthusiasm and real pleasure. Sarah, who will mind me mentioning this – but I'm the author and so outrank her – probably has the worst singing voice you have ever heard, once likened by my brother-in-law to a disgruntled sheep. Anyway, Mr Conios, Sarah's lovely class teacher, wrote in her report, 'Sarah has a lovely singing voice.' I had to take issue with him. Although I was touched by his loyalty to his charge, I felt he had gone too far in his devotion to Sarah.

Recently I corresponded with one of Sarah's inspirational teachers, Anita Brady about her days working with Sarah. 'Keeping uppermost in mind the question of how best to serve the needs of the whole child,' she wrote,

> I quickly learned the power of words. The use of positive language (referring to students who experience dyslexia or a student with Down's, rather than a dyslexic student or a Down's student) ensures we see students, like all of us, as multi-dimensional individuals with areas of strengths and weaknesses. Some see this as being pedantic or politically correct, rather than as an act of respect. As such I see a diagnosis, not as a label, but simply as a starting point from which to consider appropriate strategies to best support the individual student holistically in the here and now, and as the foundation for future growth.

We were lucky in that Sarah's presence in the classroom and, indeed the school itself, was viewed positively. It was made clear by the staff that she wasn't simply 'accepted' or 'tolerated', as they believed in the importance of embracing all and reflecting society at large. The school was quite unique in its intake, with an even spread of pupils across solidly middle-class backgrounds, refugees, and those from local estates. Children are very accepting of differences and, by being in such a mixed environment, they simply accepted each other as individual characters. That Sarah was a member of the class on a full-time basis, and not for just part of the day, was vital for her inclusion 'Classmates saw classmates struggle and succeed,' concluded Anita, 'and all students were celebrated for their success – be it baby steps or big giant steps.'

Reading this I realise how lucky we were to have teachers as dedicated, as wise as Anita, and for Sarah to be integrated into mainstream schooling, which was very important for her personal development as well as her education. This isn't, of course, the case for all children with special needs. For some parents, 'special schooling' is the right option for their children, as long as the choice is made for positive reasons and not a last resort or for want of viable alternatives.

Sarah's special needs asistant, Sarah Stubbs, remained in post since nursery, and throughout primary school, and showed herself to be utterly dedicated and committed. That continuity was also vital to Sarah's education. The two Sarahs had warmed to each other instantly, and enjoyed a very special rapport.

During this time, Sarah was enjoying a very busy social life. She was learning to swim, having sleep-overs, and loved going to the theatre. One particularly fond memory was panto at the Hackney Empire, and going backstage to see Teresa Gallagher, a lovely actress who had appeared in Sarah's radio series, and Clive Rowe 'the Dame', who let Sarah try on some of his wigs. The most delightful of men and a fabulous Dame! Sarah herself appeared in a production of *The Jungle Book* and read a joke to the whole school at assembly to raise money for Comic Relief:

'What goes ha-ha *bonk*?'

'A man laughing his head off.'

This, coincidentally, is the only joke Allie can ever remember. I just wish I'd written some better material for Sarah.

Perhaps the only slight difference of opinion with the school was when Sarah was about six. In a well-intentioned but ultimately misguided attempt to reflect Sarah's identity, in the same way it was common to have dolls representing various ethnic groups, they purchased a special doll which had Down's syndrome features. The doll's rather adult-looking physiognomy, coupled with Down's syndrome features of a protruding tongue and 'sticking-out ears', gave her a distinctly odd appearance.

At that age Sarah wouldn't have wanted or identified with a caricatured DS (Down's syndrome) doll. Allie thought it was horrible, and even overheard a teacher referring to it as 'peculiar'. 'Integration is the key to normalising Down's syndrome,' as Allie remarked, 'rather than drawing unnecessary attention to it through dolls.'

We weren't sure who these dolls were designed to help as children and since Sarah was the sole child in the school with Down's syndrome, the doll was certain to become a 'Sarah doll', and hence a caricature of her. Unless one was going to have a doll representing every child, this could only serve to introduce an unnecessarily negative image of her. Far from educating others about children with Down's syndrome, such dolls only single children like Sarah out and stereotype them just because they have the condition. We made our feelings clear that the introduction of the doll would not be beneficial to Sarah, or the other children in their understanding of her, and the whole idea was dropped.

For some reason dolls like this re-appeared in 2008, following some publicity in the national press. Some of them attempted to normalise Down's, but others were of such poor quality that they really didn't represent children with the syndrome. I'm all for anything that promotes inclusivity for children with Down's syndrome and brings them into mainstream society, but I don't think these grotesque dolls promote a positive identity or help with self-esteem.

Sarah and I subsequently appeared on *BBC Breakfast* together with a female psychologist to be interviewed by Sian Williams and Bill Turnbull on the issue. I think I was supposed to be to be speaking against the dolls, with the psychologist meant to be very pro – presumably so that a bit of an argument would ensue. In fact, neither of us could get very worked up, and the only thing we argued about was the psychologist's allegiance to Arsenal. Sarah's main objection was that the dolls were dressed in 'old-fashioned, terrible outfits.' There are lots of things to get angry about when it comes to prejudice and discrimination, but we didn't think 'Dolls with Down's' was one of them.

In September 2003 Sarah started secondary school at Alexandra Park School (APS), where I had served as a governor, helping to set up the new school. This was not so much an act of incredible selflessness and commitment, as a more self-interested involvement, in that I wanted to know what sort of school our children would be attending. I managed to inveigle myself onto the interviewing panel for the SENCO to ensure the right appointment was made. (Pauline Smith was indeed the right choice). The headteacher, Ros Hudson – a sort of very liberal Miss Jean Brodie – had said to me that she would recognise the school as a true comprehensive when Sarah walked through the gates.

On that day, Allie was at work, and Sarah wanted to walk to school on her own, but I made some excuse to accompany her, as I wanted to see her enter the school. I had tears in my eyes as she fearlessly entered the grounds and Daniel's year head, Sharon Hutchinson, spotted me and gave me a congratulatory hug. It was a wonderful moment.

Ring, Ring Goes The Bell

On the third day at APS, we received a call from the special needs assistant, informing us that Sarah would be late coming home because she had been given a detention. I hadn't signed her home/school book. Initially my reaction was one of horror – how could they do this my Sarah? She's got Down's syndrome, for goodness' sake! Surely they should make some allowances, and anyway it was my fault. Absolutely ridiculous! But then Allie and talked about it and we realised the school was quite right: in some ways Sarah had to be treated like everyone else, and it was the correct thing to do. She was completely fine about it, but when she got home, gave me a ticking off for being 'a hopeless dad'.

Daniel had been at the school for two years, and Allie was initially worried that he would now feel responsible for protecting Sarah, and that it might hold him back both socially and academically. In fact, in the early days he did want to walk to school with her, but she wanted to be independent and refused. (Daniel later put this down to his 'tardiness and lack of enthusiasm in the mornings', and the fact that she 'revelled in the independence of being first out the door and taking her own route.')

Sarah did indeed love school, and couldn't wait to get there in the morning. Her reading was great; her maths was terrible. She was always the first in the school to volunteer for anything, no matter what it entailed. It was all something of a party for her. Lucy Parry was one of Sarah's teachers, and I asked her for some memories of their time together.

> When I think of Sarah the following memories of her charming, loving, strong, and very occasionally exasperating, personality come up!
>
> When I first started working with Sarah she wanted to show me her dance moves, so she and

Alison invited me round after school one day. After Sarah pointed me out to her mum – 'She's my friend, not yours' – she took me up to her room and said squarely, pointing at the bed, 'You, sit there,' as she shook her hair free and then started dancing about her room. This delighted me then, and still makes me smile – her bossiness, her openness, and complete lack of self-consciousness due to her love of dancing. She was the star of her own show; I saw myself reflected in her. I loved her wilfulness and sense of fun and life . . . She is utterly unique.

Lucy recalled the fun they had during a lesson in the library one day as they shared the Welsh legend of Gelert:

Sarah listened with total attention, acting out the actions for each part, whether it was Llewelyn's beloved hound fighting the wolf, defending the baby prince in the cradle, or Llewelyn's grief at discovering he'd mistakenly slain his favourite hound. . . Sarah brought the scene to life with feeling and animation – the librarian who was working around us was so moved by the scene we created. Sarah brought the force of her personality to all she did, livening up teaching and learning for all involved! Thank goodness!

It was in one of our lessons in the library that I told Sarah I'd be leaving the school that half-term. Sarah challenged me initially.

'No, you can't – who'll take me out of French? Miss Madame Smith [Sarah always referred to her

French teacher by both titles, as we still do] says I come to you during French.'

When I said again that arrangements would be made for her French, she opened her school planner and started to write to a note for her mum saying that I was leaving. She spoke as she wrote: 'Dear Mum, Miss Parry says she is leaving' – and then she put her head on the desk and cried. Ahh! – this broke my heart! I went home with a cracking headache, and had to lie down and have a cry too. This is the power of Sarah – her honesty, her vibrancy and fullness of being, together with an open and warm heart, is so deeply touching, cracking open the hearts of others around her. May she continue to do this, because it is much needed. In my 21 years of teaching, Sarah is still my most memorable student, which makes her very special.

Although she attended mainstream school, most of Sarah's friends around this time did have learning difficulties. It was difficult for her to be close to other 13- and 14-year-old girls, because they can be so sophisticated. In year 9, for example, a group of girls got her to dance provocatively, filmed it and uploaded it to *YouTube*. The offending material was discovered very quickly and removed, and the girls were excluded temporarily. I asked the headmistress if I could see these girls and have a quiet word with them, but Ros, thinking I might do more than whisper in their shell-likes, declined my offer. Very sensible – I guess that's why she was the Head. In fact, that incident was the only bullying Sarah ever experienced throughout all her school and college years. She's been lucky, as over 80 per cent of young people with a learning disability have experienced bullying. If you have a learning disability you are twice as likely to be bullied as other children. Despite the fact that the internet has been a powerful force for progress in terms of support, education and information, attacks on people with disabilities are commonly posted on *YouTube* as so called 'entertainment.'

Thanks to Sarah we have come to know so many people that we would never have met, and found ourselves in worlds previously unknown to us. In September 2007, we attended a reception at 10 Downing Street, given by Sarah Brown to raise awareness about Down's syndrome. The building is something of a Tardis, in that it appears small from the exterior but, once inside, corridors and hallways lead into more and more rooms and floors. On ascending the stairs, we passed General Petraeus and other US Army top brass huddled in a corner, and we were then led into one of the main reception rooms.

The staff were surprisingly relaxed, and let us explore the Cabinet Office and other rooms. Naturally all the guests were wondering if the then Prime Minister, Gordon Brown, was nearby, but no-one dared enquire his whereabouts – apart from Sarah, who marched straight up to her namesake and asked, 'Is Gordon here?' Sarah Brown was amused, and replied that he was somewhere in the building, although we never clapped eyes on him. I was very impressed with Sarah Brown, who was quite at ease with the children and adults with Down's, and before she officially welcomed the attendees we had a chat with her. When it came to her prepared speech she included some of our conversation – she had clearly been listening carefully to some of our gripes.

In December the following year we went to a Christmas carol service at Normansfield, where there was an auction for Spice

Girls concert tickets. We bid (I have to admit somewhat half-heartedly), and we were outbid by the actress Emma Barton, who is a patron of the DSA. However, Emma very kindly gave the tickets to Sarah, who was thrilled. Subsequently she wrote about her experience:

> When I went to see the spice girls concert live in O2 Arena I was totally having fun I was screaming out loud and was waving my phone around and I couldn't believe that I was in the VIP lounge I was extreemly excited About the whole thing I told everyone at school They were jealos. that was the best Thing happened to me in 2008 on the day before my birthday and on my birthday I got the spice girls cd. I love them! Someday I want to meet them in person and get Autographs
>
> Thank you all for doing this to me I am a very grateful person.

SARAH MERRIMAN AGED 16

One of the most important, continuing activities that Sarah pursued for ten years during this time was a dance and movement class that involved about ten young people with Down's. Run as a weekly session by Sara Bannerman, an ex-dancer and innovative chorographer, not only did it deliver a creative outlet for Sarah, but it also provided her with a group of friends with whom she is still in touch. Let Sarah explain:

> I really enjoyed the dance groups because I can see all my friends there it was awesome over the years and

now we are all grownups. There was Annalie, because I have known her since I was born she is fantastic and lovely my closest friend. Jess is great, the first person with Down's syndrome that mum and dad ever knew, Ophir is wonderful and really pretty she's great friend as well. Then Hannah she is totally awesome and funny that's what I like about her. Raffy he always makes me Laugh he is a joker I like that about him he's cool dude. Max the biggest star there. . . he appeared in a film. And Robbie he is totally cool and funny and he supports West Ham! Nikita she is way cool and she makes me laugh. Jonathon he is new to the group and he likes to play football and he is a lovely friend and Victoria she is so sweet and lovely she is cool. I think Sara is great because she gives us tips about dancing. She has been a brilliant teacher to us for ten years.

Both Daniel and younger brother Joel volunteered to help with the group, which became known as 'Dance and Drama' – Joel recalls the emphasis as being sometimes more on the drama. Most of them wanted to be the star of the show, and there was a lot of backstage rivalry, resulting in bickering, arguments, hiding under tables, and tears. Not unlike any other group of performers.

But as the years passed they matured into a cohesive troupe who all got on well – unlike some other performers. Sara was incredibly patient, but firm when she needed to be, and gave the participants the improvisational freedom to express their creativity, and under her guidance they produced some lovely innovative performances. It was wonderful to see the enthusiasm and warmth with which they greeted each other each week – such was the screaming and whooping with joy it was as though they hadn't clapped eyes on one another for months. Inevitably there was much hugging. I tried to instil some of this excitement in the other parents, but we just didn't have the spontaneity and joie de vivre of our kids.

The occasional romance would blossom, even if it was more imagined than real. Robbie proposed to Annalie, although his mum reminded him that it was customary for the couple to have dated at least once before an offer of marriage was made. Sarah occasionally announced that she had a boyfriend, but often failed to inform the boy in question. Max, who had just appeared with Cate Blanchett in *Notes on a Scandal*, once announced that he had two girlfriends, 'Cate Blanchett and Sarah Merriman'.

I told Sarah I didn't want her to play second fiddle to anyone, even a Hollywood star, although my words weren't heeded when she went to a birthday party and returned home very excited stating, 'We've officially hugged!'

When Sarah was about 11, she began to be aware that she had Down's, and realised herself that this was why it took her longer to learn things. She used to say she had 'funny eyes', and 'Tennis isn't my game 'cos of Down's.' We obviously tried to help her with this, but she was also cute enough to use it as an excuse, and went through a phase of trying to use it to her advantage.

'Sarah, could you please go upstairs and fetch your shoes?'
'No, I can't, I've got Downs syndrome.'

'Sarah, could you empty the dishwasher?'
'No. You know why. Down's syndrome.'

A Major Adjustment

'Turn your music down!'

'Sorry. . . Down's syndrome.'

Well, of course, we didn't stand for that – although the music never seemed to be turned down. To be honest, Sarah never gave us any trouble, and, apart from the occasional dramatic outburst, she was not a difficult teenager.

Sarah continued happily at APS, receiving three hours a week in support from a specialist teacher and 20 hours a week support from a teaching assistant, Lisa Clarke, whom Sarah adored, to assist the class teacher in the implementation of the individual programmes. 'There were many reasons to admire Sarah,' Lisa recalls.

> In spite of having learning difficulties she tried her best in any given subject. She had fantastic manners, a sense of fun, and she possessed a remarkable confidence and maturity in social situations for someone of her age. Being a teenager, there were the obvious fall-outs/fall-ins with peers and 'OMG' dramas too. However, most of all it was Sarah's fearlessness which was so impressive. She participated in all school activities – sports day was way outside her comfort zone, but she ran for all she was worth!'

Sarah received speech and language therapy, and her therapist was probably the strictest of the various professionals in tow:

> Sarah can sometimes show frustration if she perceives a task too difficult, and can refuse help from staff. When she is frustrated she can be rude to those trying

to help her, but will immediately apologise for her actions. . . Sarah continues to present with severe difficulties, which impact on her ability to follow longer and more complex instructions.

Sarah's reading skills were always her strongest - she was very keen to remind all of us that she had read *To Kill a Mockingbird*, and would be able to deliver the odd Shakespeare quotation, although she did need help with comprehension. She continued to experience difficulties with the correct use of lower and upper-case letters – and still does. Her numeracy skills improved, and in May 2008 Sarah received the Year 11 Director of Studies award, as a reward for being 'a diligent and positive member of the Year Group throughout her time at Alexandra Park School'. Her formal schooling ended with the end of year 'prom' on a boat on the Thames in the company of a very sweet boy called Jerome.

A couple of months later, in the same way as thousands of other students across the nation, Sarah went off to school to collect her GCSE results. Allie was at work, and I waited somewhat impatiently for her return. After what seemed a very long time, the doorbell rang and I rushed to the front door. There was a beaming Sarah, with a smile as broad as the Pacific Ocean across her face. 'I did it, Dad! I did it!'

Sarah had achieved the equivalent of four GCSE level passes.

7

FAMILY MATTERS

Meanwhile
Her so beguiling smile
Belies the fears
Of later years
And though we can't forget
The future isn't yet.
We must not think ahead
Instead
Enjoy her as she is
Uncork the fizz
For here's my simple toast
To Sarah
Who's fairer
And rarer
Than most.

Eric Merriman (with apologies to Ogden Nash)

Minor Adjustment, the Radio 4 comedy-drama, was quite a family affair.

I had begun writing with my father a few years previously, and he had been a well-established comedy writer for many years, having created and written for Tommy Cooper, Dave Allen, Morecambe and Wise and many others too humorous to mention.

Family Matters

Initially, the principal motivation for writing the show was simply professional: an attempt to combine humour and drama. Whilst we were addressing a serious subject, it was not meant to be a show about Down's syndrome, and we were certainly desperate to avoid being preachy or patronising the audience. But of course if the dramatic text provided some information and, more importantly, exploded some of the myths, about Down's syndrome, then this would be an added bonus.

The producer Gareth Edwards came up with the idea of having Sarah, then aged five, in the show to play the part of Amy, as he thought it would create a family atmosphere in the studio. Sarah had her very own professional chaperone in the form of my mother, Jean Merriman, who had worked in this field for many years. And Daniel even played a cameo role as a 'spoilt child' – not type-casting, I have to say. . .

All the cast were wonderfully kind and patient with Sarah, and Samantha Bond, who had two small children at the time, spent a lot of time playing with and reading to Sarah. Indeed, she actually insisted on Sarah being in a number of scenes that we hadn't written her into. By the end of the series Sarah was extraordinarily confident, and on the day of the last recording strode into the studio, theatrically threw her bag on to the nearest chair, and announced her arrival with a 'Hello everyone, I'm here.'

Once the project was in production, it seemed to develop a life of its own, and the show created a great deal of media interest. Sarah, Peter Davison and I were also asked to appear on the *Good Morning* show with Richard Madeley and Judy Finnegan. Shortly after, Allie, myself, Daniel and Sarah were interviewed on the *After 5* programme by Caron Keating, the daughter of Gloria Hunniford, who died from cancer in 2004 at the age of 41.

A Major Adjustment

On the way home, the driver who collected us from the television studio told us that the previous day Marlon Brando had been a passenger in his car.

'Bit of a comedown for you to drive us now,' I told him.

'Not really,' he said. 'He's just another client and . . . in any case your family are a lot easier on my suspension.'

The whole experience of being involved in *Minor Adjustment* was quite marvellous, and very exciting for all the family. I hadn't realised that writing the show would be such a cathartic experience, and I was able to laugh and joke about things with my dad that would have been impossible when Sarah was born. At that time, I had neither wanted nor felt the need to bare my soul, but by looking at another family, albeit of our creation, I found I was projecting my own thoughts and feelings into their fictitious personae and in turn reflecting on how I felt. I was so proud of Sarah, and at the end of the series Gareth Edwards bought her a present and sent her a card which read, 'Here's a big "Thank You" to one of the most professional actresses we've ever worked with.' It would also be true to say that she was probably the only one who wasn't potty-trained.

In January 1996, Sarah was a bridesmaid at the wedding of Gareth and Frances Wedgwood. We were greatly touched that Sarah should be so honoured, but also, due to the conventions of the occasion, slightly wary of other people's reactions to her and what they might think. Would they realise that Sarah had Down's syndrome, and what, if anything, would it mean to them? Did we want to announce it to all up front so that any errant behaviour might be excused, or should we just keep quiet and let her be herself? We needn't have worried. Everyone at this rather grand affair was extremely kind and thoughtful, and the two adult bridesmaids looked after Sarah admirably.

It was quite a coincidence that we had cast Peter Davison as Sarah's father for his skill and professionalism, only to discover that he was actually a patron of the DSA and had a cousin, Linda, with Down's, who had died at the age of 40 from heart disease. We have stayed in touch with Peter, and I worked with him on his recent autobiography *Is There Life Outside The Box?* I took Sarah to see him backstage when he was appearing in *Legally Blonde* at the Savoy Theatre, and he very kindly organised some autographs for her and sent an email the following day: 'I can't tell you how lovely it was to see you and Sarah last night. She is every bit as sweet and beautiful as she was all those years ago.'

From the beginning we had incredible support and love from our parents and relatives. Allie's father, John Wellemin, who was born in Prague, fled to England before the war, and many more of his family were wiped out by the Nazis. John returned to Prague with the Czech army after the war, but escaped from the Communists in 1948 and eventually settled in England, where he met Ursula at a language school. Although not an outwardly emotional man, his contribution to *A Minor Adjustment* was very touching, especially when describing his feelings immediately after Sarah's birth:

> Certainly we did not feel there was much to cele-
> brate. . . I talked to my wife with forced joviality, not
> daring to mention the fears all of us had for the future.
> I had the desire to talk to someone freely about my
> real concerns and, as I did so often, I sat down at my
> computer to write to my best friend Honza in Prague
> to whom I opened my heart; this made me feel more
> composed.

A Major Adjustment

What had struck me most over the first few months of Sarah's life was the obvious love Daniel displayed towards his sister. The tenderness with which he treated her surprised me. When a similar tenderness was shown also by Sarah's cousins, Tom and Nick, I started wondering whether these very young children had an instinct that made them feel Sarah needed even more support than other babies. Most of the time when I am with Sarah I am oblivious that she has Down's syndrome as she is just my beloved granddaughter, Sarah. Yet the concern about how Sarah will develop over the next few decades . . . as a grandfather my greatest concern is that she should be happy whatever level of achievement she attains.

John had no reason to worry about her development and achievements, and would be so proud of his 'beloved granddaughter, Sarah'. He died in 2006 following a long illness with cancer, and Sarah remembers 'Pop John' with great fondness, singing Czech songs to her at bedtime and teaching her to play tennis.

Sarah has fond memories of her other grandfather, 'Grandpa Eric', when we used to holiday in Suffolk, 'when he used to make me laugh and buying me treats.' My dad died in June 2003, and for a comedy writer his deathbed scene was completely apt. A junior doctor, attempting some kind of counselling, had previously asked Dad how he would feel if the treatment didn't work. 'Dead!' was the immediate response. However, Dad's consultant for many years was a brilliant surgeon, an ex-Guards officer and something of a maverick, with a bluff, jovial manner that Dad appreciated. Mum and I were called up to the hospital early one morning with the news that Dad wasn't expected to live much longer. Half an hour later we stood behind the closed curtains around the bed, where Dad lay unconscious. The end was inevitable. The consultant then arrived with his entourage, greeted us warmly, and delivered a rousing speech along the lines of, 'Well, it looks grim, but he's comfortable and we're doing all that we can. He's a strong chap and. . .'

The ward sister nudged me and whispered, 'I'm afraid your father has passed away.'

The consultant didn't seem to notice Dad's demise, and continued in full pomp: 'Anyway, we'll see what we can do. . . You never quite know what the future holds, and he's still fighting. . .' With that, and hearty handshakes for us both, he departed.

As sad as Mum and I were, we couldn't help but think that this was such a fitting end for a comedy writer. Dad would have appreciated it - although he might have written a different 'tag'.

When we told Sarah about Dad's death, her immediate response was, 'I'm too shocked to cry.' She recovered herself to ask me some months later if I missed my dad. I said I did, and her response was, 'But you've got him in your heart . . . and on video.' Sarah still talks about him an awful lot, as she does about her maternal grandfather. In fact, she still becomes very sad and tearful about her grandfathers as though they have passed away just a few days previously, and care staff who don't know her that well sometimes show great empathy and understanding at her sorrowful mood, and ring us to offer condolences and inquire whether Sarah needs extra support.

'Oh, no need to worry,' we explain cheerfully. 'The grandfathers died years ago – she's fine.' Some must think we're very callous but, although we're sympathetic, we don't always indulge her.

There is mutual love and devotion between our mothers and

Sarah. 'Over five years ago when you were born,' wrote Allie's mother, Ursula, a Jewish refugee from Germany, in *A Minor Adjustment*,

> and we heard that you had Down's syndrome, we were not happy. You were not what we expected, and we did not know how you were going to develop. Things have changed so much since those anxious times immediately after your birth. We have seen you grow up and develop, and watched all the improvements with great pleasure. We are so happy with you, our lovely granddaughter. The description that fits you is 'charming', a word that is not usually in my vocabulary, but you inspire me to use it. Don't let this go to your head.

I'm glad it hasn't for the most part, and it's borne out by Ursula's more recent words:

> Since that time, 18 years ago, Sarah has blossomed into an even more confident, self-assured adult. Throughout her life the people she has been in contact with have been special. Could this be that she is a magnet that attracts the best people? I am so proud and happy about all Sarah's public achievements, and even more so about her progress and lovely personality.

My mother had found Sarah's birth particularly difficult, and secretly she was suffering:

I felt that I needed to show strength and indeed encouragement to Andrew, Alison, and of course to my first grandchild, Daniel, on whom I doted. I wanted them to know that they had my whole-hearted support. It was especially difficult for me since I had always had two great fears where babies were concerned. Cot deaths and Down's syndrome. Both now haunted me. I lost our second son, Christopher, in a cot death at nine months. And here was the second 'tragedy'. Lightning had struck twice.

Now she feels very differently.

Sarah has exceeded all my hopes and expectations. The way things have turned out is no small thanks to the love and support of her parents and her two brothers. I love spending time with her, she is an amazing young woman, full of life and purpose. I am so proud of her – if only her grandfathers could see her now. My goodness, how very happy and thankful they would be.

My mum celebrated her 90th birthday last year, and Sarah gave the following speech.

So Grandma this is your day to celebrate your birthday. Enjoy every minute of it. Just a few words I would like to say about my Grandma. You are amazing and a big part of my life and you've been such a wonderful grandma in the whole wide world!

Let's enjoy it with all your family and friends and granddaughter and grandsons – and son – that's Andy (sorry, grandma that's Andrew to you) my dad and cousins.

So happy birthday, grandma. Love you!

Sarah has had a huge impact on her siblings, which has in turn shaped their life philosophy and future careers. They have both volunteered to work with children and adults with learning disabilities. When Daniel was a child, we asked him if he minded that Sarah had Down's syndrome. 'No,' he replied, 'because I love her.' He also once said that he was glad he didn't have Down's syndrome, because 'I might be like Sarah and she can be really annoying.'

All siblings have feelings of jealousy and rivalry, and we all know how such feelings can be brought to the fore by the arrival of a new baby, who will inevitably need a lot of attention. But when a new baby like Sarah joins the family, the effect on existing siblings can be quite profound. The necessity of being open and honest with Daniel had to be counterbalanced with care that he not be overburdened with what can easily become a family obsession. From a very early age, however, Daniel found Sarah's presence very comforting. When he was met by Allie and Sarah at the end of his day at nursery he used to go straight up to Sarah and stroke her face for a few minutes before he would consider leaving the school premises. He was always incredibly affectionate towards her.

'There is no evidence that having a [Down's syndrome] child in the family automatically produces ill-effects in the other children', writes Cliff Cunningham in his book *Down's Syndrome: An Introduction for Parents*. 'In fact there is evidence that many families gain from the experience.' The general feeling of parents is that their other children are not adversely affected by having a sibling with Down's syndrome. In fact, it seems, the experience of having a sibling with a disability can make them more mature, sensitive and considerate. Daniel does seem to understand Sarah better than anybody, and was always generally quite tolerant of her ways and foibles. Of course, their relationship is by no means one-sided – it is actually quite symbiotic. Research has shown that a sibling can enhance the social environment of a disabled child, and thus have a positive effect on his or her progress.

There are, of course, great difficulties in any sibling relationship, and obvious and not so obvious traps one can fall into. For example, there was a tendency to let Sarah get away with things: it wasn't that her behaviour was bad: it was that she didn't understand what she was being told. The notion that his sister was not a 'naughty girl', but rather a 'Down's girl', and therefore not totally responsible for her behaviour, cut no ice with Daniel – and still doesn't.

Here is Daniel himself on life with Sarah.

> Everything should be prefaced with the fact I don't really know life without Sarah. She's my sister two years junior, and we're close enough in age that she's always seen her birthdays as one step closer to finally catching me up. The relationship has always felt different to that with my younger brother Joel, to whom sibling competition seemed to transfer. Given the arguments we used to have – usually fashioned by myself – it's quite possible that I bottled up a need for an outpouring of elder-brother superiority for a few years later, as this was never a facet of my relationship with Sarah.

A Major Adjustment

I'll never know how much a lack of sibling rivalry with Sarah in the traditional sense has to do with Down's. Joel came to the party a bit later, once Sarah and I were already such a team. When our parents were away, it was never me babysitting the other two, as Sarah didn't allow it. It was us in charge of Joel. All I know is that by way of her determination and sheer gregariousness, Sarah has refused to ever accept second place, and has earned this status in the family and wider world.

When the attention around the radio show and previous book was in full swing, it was great fun to be part of it all. TV and press coverage were the norm, and naturally Sarah was at the centre of it. Sarah signing a pile of her books three times her height, with her glasses at the end of her nose, became a routine sight in the kitchen. It was a big deal to be featured in the *Radio Times* in those days, and I didn't bat an eyelid at a feature in the *Daily Mail* or having my painting of Sarah reproduced in the *Guardian*.

Apparently, this 'all eyes on Sarah' stage was consuming our family life to the extent that I deserved a PlayStation. I couldn't work out why mum and dad felt it necessary to remind me that I hadn't been forgotten by buying me a games console, but I wasn't going to complain. I understand this now as a classic parental concern: all the attention was on the new sibling on the block, and with added media interest, and they must have been wary about me feeling left out. It didn't feel this way, and my cameo in episode 6 of *Minor Adjustment*, and a place on the sofa live on

ITV, were just the start of unheralded exposure to riches that would have been denied in an alternative universe of having a 'typical' sis.

Around then it already went without saying that Sarah just needed – and merited – a little more attention, and it has felt so ever since. Whether that has been help with something like maths, or people regularly wanting to know how she's doing, the outside interest Sarah has attracted has therefore gone hand-in-hand with who she is, and has become part of who we are. Sarah is merely part of the fabric – otherwise, to think about the impact of Sarah's disability actually takes conscious work and deep introspection. I believe that the 'adjustment' has been more my parents' to make. To me, having Sarah as my sister is second nature.

I've loved including Sarah in my social life wherever possible. It's easy. She's come to my birthday house parties, and we've gone out clubbing – there's no chance that only my younger brother would be invited. Transport and arrangements need more attention to detail, but that's no reason to exclude her, and she's always a hit. Sarah is infamous for going backstage after a performance and telling each actor or entertainer that she meets in turn that they were her particular favourite. There's no guile intended: she just wants everyone to feel special. While holidaying in Santa Monica, we all went to Magicopolis, a theatre for magic events and entertainment. At the end of the show, when all the magicians came into the foyer to meet the audience, Sarah shamelessly went up to each 'act' and told them, 'You were the best!'

And when we went clubbing, each of my 'DJ-ing' mates were her favourites. She remembers everyone's names, and is uncanny in knowing what people want to hear about and what they want to be asked about. Of course, there are some people she does not click with. Not everyone 'gets' her, and likewise she is also discriminating. Nevertheless, she takes people to heart like nobody's business. The teachers and her assistants at school would become fast favourites, whilst those who moved on would never be forgotten. She is acutely aware of those who value her, and she reciprocates. There has never been any hesitation introducing her to friends, or worrying about their reactions. Quite the opposite, in fact.

In *A Minor Adjustment*, when I was seven, I wrote as one of my main aims for Sarah that I'd one day like to go with her to a football match, and this is now one of my favourite things to do with her. I was watching the build-up to a north London derby on TV once, and Sarah could be seen full-view in our front-row seats at the corner flag of the old White Hart Lane, screaming profanities at Robin van Persie in a previous match against Arsenal. She's thrown one of her Spurs shirts in the bin after one acrimonious cup defeat too many, and has enjoyed meeting a few players.

It is fortunate that our football tastes align, because our musical tastes certainly don't. Sarah rarely veers outside the mainstream packaged pop sphere, much to the dismay of Joel and me. Sarah will forever be a teenybopper, and this also goes for her taste in TV, film and most popular culture, which remains incredibly Disney-centric, and is probably what I see as one of the most identifiable manifestations of her immaturity. One saving grace is that her knowledge of film and TV casts is akin to having a human IMDB for a sister. Something I also wrote in *A Minor Adjustment* was that if Sarah was a Spice Girl she'd be 'Spaghetti Spice', which I guess I maintain. Certainly, truth be told, going to the Spice Girls musical *Viva Forever* was one of the more difficult older-brother things I have done with Sarah. Everything else has been a breeze in comparison.

I recall frustrations at a certain point when my parents seemed to regard Sarah as almost the finished article much earlier than Joel and me. It started to feel like Sarah's foibles (so stubborn sometimes) would be dismissed or ignored when ours were not, and Sarah was of course still capable of improvement and exceeding expectations. I guess it came with her development having been considered as no longer such a concern, and when she had achieved a certain level of independence, which when she was born was never guaranteed. It is also equally likely that these frustrations came from that familiar trait of older siblings feeling their younger ones get a better deal.

I'm aware of someone with Down's having passed their driving test, but it would not be right for Sarah. She's pretty much mastered the bus routes, and has also proved herself on the Tube. I have to admit that I once lost her on the Piccadilly line on the way to meet one of our grandmothers at the Royal Academy. Sarah tends to walk slightly more slowly than me, and as the doors opened on the train I jumped on, thinking Sarah was closer behind me. The doors shut, and Sarah was behind the glass. I madly gestured to stay where she was, as I intended to come back as soon as I could, but it must have looked like nonsense. I should have been horrified with myself, but I kind of had faith she wouldn't do anything silly, and would approach a member of staff if need be.

I got off at the next stop and returned to where we had separated. No sign. I got off again at the next stop in case she had misread my wild gestures. Still no sign. I did start to worry at this point, although my main concern was that Sarah would plainly never let me forget this (once reunited), especially given that I had done this to her on her birthday of all days. I left the train at Green Park in a panic and called Grandma. 'Are you with Sarah?' I asked hurriedly.

I received a confused 'No' in reply, as *I* was supposed to be with her. Sarah did not answer her mobile. I carried on to the Royal Academy, and planned to try and locate her from there somehow. I would also have a justifiably worried grandmother to contend with. When I arrived in the forecourt Sarah was there, and gave me one hell of a look – a hell of a look I was happy to see. We had never mentioned exactly where we were going, but Green Park must have been said in passing, and this was enough for her to find the gallery and Grandma without me.

Some years later, I took Sarah to Paris once for a weekend, as a trip on the Eurostar had always been something she wanted to do, given she is not too keen on flying. We stayed in the city in a cheap hotel and she loved the urban buzz and noise of the traffic in the 7ᵉ Arrondissement. She's a proper city girl. We did so much walking, and enjoyed the cafés, crepes, and escargots. Sadly, it wouldn't be possible for Sarah to do this trip with a friend or boyfriend. She goes on organised trips once or twice a year, and on family holidays, but to 'up sticks' and traverse unknown territories is beyond her and, to my mind, one of life's great joys.

I feel an immediate affinity with those whose lives have been touched by intellectual disability, and often need to suppress the urge to engage in a knowing nod when chancing upon people and their families/friends with Down's. Such inclination towards the world of DS has led me to quite a few exploits: fundraising for the Down's Syndrome Association, volunteering with children with disabilities in India in a classic gap year endeavour, and I believe it must also have informed (at least in part) my choice of career in law, as a representative for the voiceless and vulnerable in immigration/asylum and human rights cases.

Joel and I don't think about Sarah's future too much. Things have gone swimmingly for Sarah, but then our parents do what needs to be done. If she wasn't independent, things would be different, but we will have our role to play. It is well known that Sarah has an increased risk to many life-limiting conditions compared to Joel and me, but this is a bridge that is to be crossed when we come to it. Such challenges will be broached as and when, as they have been throughout Sarah's life. We just hope that the mixture of fortune and circumstance that has held us in good stead continues to do so. There's nothing else to it. Whether it should or not, her future feels far from anything remotely chipping away at me at this point.

Such concerns lie more with the case of people with Down's in general. At the same time as people with the disability appear to be breaking ground in ways truly unforeseen – running marathons, teaching education programmes, Ted-EX talks, speeches to Congress, presenting the news, owning businesses, lifting world cups (Álvaro, the son of the victorious Spanish manager in 2010, Vicente del Bosque, has DS and participated in the team's celebrations) – you also have the prospect of a similar breakthrough altogether more dark: that of fully 'Down's syndrome-free' nations. It is terrifying, and a real fork in the road. It feels that it is up to people like us to show the value of people like Sarah to wider society in terms that transcend eugenics/Darwinism and zero-sum economics. Only then can parents make an informed choice.

I'm a very passive and tranquil person. I have never been in a fight. I've often thought, however, that if someone said something out of turn to or about Sarah – whoever they were – I would lose my cool. This has not happened, but remains possible. People use the terms 'retard', and the more problematic 'Mong', in common parlance. I correct people, but don't risk things tipping over. It can also feel hypocritical. Do I correct 'Spazzy'? I try to and find that there is reasoning to be done in some instances, yet not in others. These are terms used generally, and not aimed at Sarah or her contemporaries, but the implications are there.

Your turn, Joel. . .

When asked to contribute to *A Major Adjustment*, I still felt aggrieved that my dad had not given me the opportunity to inscribe my initial thoughts about Sarah for *A Minor Adjustment*. Though only two years old at the time, I already had much to say. Anyway, after countless meetings with my manager, my people in Hollywood, my agent and the author, I finally consented to write a passage. After all, they are family. Furthermore, my birth had owed much to the extra chromosome – Sarah had been a pivotal part of the very conscious decision to bring me into the world.

The third child (me) was not of course to replace Sarah, but for Mum to experience a birth that was somewhat less dramatic than the last. Bringing me into the world would also lessen the 'burden' for Daniel, in terms of providing support for Sarah when my parents got older. I'm more than happy to fulfil that role, although with Sarah becoming increasingly independent I'm not sure that I will be needed. Despite my being born with one less chromosome than Sarah, God knows what the doctor would have said about me if they had possessed a crystal ball; 'Well, he will be able to walk and talk, but I'm not sure obtaining an arts degree will ever give him an opportunity to contribute to society. I'm afraid he's going to be a burden. . .' With Sarah's career going from strength to strength, it will be me who will be WhatsApping my big sister in 30 years asking if she could pay my gas bill.

As we've both lived away from home in recent years, Sarah's recent installation of WhatsApp has enabled us to keep in touch over social media, albeit in a very sporadic and disjointed away, in great contrast to the repartee we share in person. Usually I'll get a message from Sarah saying, 'I miss you', or 'How's Norwich mate?' – when I've actually been studying in America. Admittedly, this was only once, and when I reminded her I was in a vegan bakery in San Francisco and not in Gregg's on Colman Road, she instantly remembered where I was.

It is indeed Sarah who is more on the ball than me about remembering certain events, often reminding me on WhatsApp about specific family anniversaries that I may have forgotten. With Daniel and Sarah both being older than me, I could always look to them for tastes in movies, food and music. Well, perhaps more from Daniel. This was not only because of the male influence, but also because S Club 7 never really tickled my fancy. Shy as a child, I was always amazed at the enthusiasm and exuberance Sarah would show at social events, when she'd fearlessly stroll up to people she didn't know and introduce herself – a gift with which any adult would be comfortable. What was equally special was that the person she'd usually start talking to would instantly take to her within seconds. It is the constant positive energy that she can exert on others when participating in the most mundane tasks as well as in social occasions, which endlessly amazes me.

Though the attendees at the Dance and Drama group, which Dad wrote about in a previous chapter, may not have been the most articulate, one word in their vocabulary that was certainly absent was 'prejudice'. I honestly believe that had ET walked into Alexandra Palace Community centre at 5.30 p.m. on a Monday night, the first question they'd have asked the Extra-Terrestrial would have been, 'Have you got the new Hannah Montana CD?'

What amazes me is that societal norms and constructions do not bother Sarah and her friends one bit. The family were recently at our cousin's wedding, and Sarah shook a leg on her own on the dance floor. The funny thing is the other guests were all at the bar getting drinks, while Sarah didn't need one drop of alcohol. The lack of self-consciousness in a society that pathologises any kind of difference, and expects perfection, is simply admirable. I sometimes hear people say that this person or that 'suffers with Down's Syndrome', but I can guarantee that in Sarah's case, such people are suffering more than her.

There are occasions when siblings will not admit that they have a brother or sister who has special needs. Not because they may be embarrassed by their disability, but because they don't necessarily want to have to explain what is wrong with their family member. There are also siblings who might be embarrassed at having friends home to play. This was never the case with Daniel or Joel's friends, who without exception are genuinely fond of Sarah.

I shocked my three 'kids' a couple of years ago when I said I wasn't at all interested in having grandchildren, and, although I would be delighted for them, don't expect me to play a part. I'd witnessed friends and acquaintances used and abused by their children by being inveigled into hours of cheap childcare – not even allowed to take holidays as it would interfere with their precious grandchildren's routines. I'd changed nappies for nearly 15 years when they were younger, and I wasn't doing that again. And as for feeding ducks with clinging toddlers, or pushing them endlessly on swings and making polite conversation with equally bored grandparents – well, please include me out. All you hear from exploited grandparents is that it's great because you can give the children back at the end of the day. If it's so wonderful to hand them back to their parents, why look after them in the first place?

In fact, the only kids I'm interested in now are those who have Down's syndrome. It's true that our family have become a little obsessed with children and adults with Down's syndrome. Allie, who is now at the stage where babies and toddlers hold little interest, still comes over all soppy and maternal in the company of a young child with Down's syndrome. As she related earlier, at a DSA conference crèche she came close to an out-of-body experience.

If I see a person with Down's syndrome I want to know all about him or her: their story; what they do; who their people are. Once, at a wedding, Daniel and I spotted someone in a pushchair who we thought was a toddler with DS. We stared at him from all angles, indulged ourselves in whispered discussion, weighed up all the possibilities without having the confidence to make an approach. It was only when Dan and I shyly introduced ourselves that we discovered Sarah had already accosted the child's mother and asked, 'Has he got Down's syndrome like me?' He did have Down's, and his mum was charmed by Sarah's confident and no-nonsense approach. Family means everything to Sarah, as demonstrated in this birthday card to Allie's sister, Carey.

> Have a great Birthday you're the best auntie I have got. I hope your birthday bash went well? Your been a star to me Thanks for being There since I was a baby your sister is very kind to you always because she's my mum. And Carey I am very proud of you and I am glad to be your neice Hugs and kisses love Sarah

We celebrated Sarah's own landmark 18th birthday in 2010 with a party at the house. We invited family, friends and some of the professionals who had helped her and us throughout the years. Daniel (keyboards), Joel (guitar and vocals) and cousin Tom (piano) formed a band for the evening with my dear mate Danny (alto saxophone). They are still awaiting offers to perform a second gig. . .

In July 2016 Joel went to study for a year in California at San Francisco State University. Sarah sent a heartfelt text: 'I'm going to miss him so much its not like a family any more we are having separate lives.'

8

ART AND SOUL

The true artist will let his wife starve, his children go barefoot, his mother drudge for his living at 70, sooner than work at anything but his art.

George Bernard Shaw

In the enlightening *New Approaches to Down Syndrome*, Brian Stratford discusses artists of the Renaissance, and describes how Andrea Mantegna (1431–1506) was one of the first artists to use living people as models for his paintings. One of his works, *Madonna and Child*, is exhibited at the Uffizi museum in Florence. It was created whilst he was the court painter for the rich and powerful Gonzaga family in 15th-century Mantua, and the child undoubtedly has Down's syndrome. Angels surrounding the *Madonna della Humilita* painted about 1437 by the Carmelite friar Filippo Lippi have certain characteristics of Down's syndrome, and the Flemish artist Jacob Jordaens (1593–1678) had a daughter with Down's syndrome who featured in some of his paintings.

In more recent times, the subject has become the artist, as the paintbrush has been passed on to a number of talented painters and illustrators with Down's. One of the first I met was Sally Johnson, an enigmatic, extraordinary woman – and yet her birth, in 1974, was greeted with total negativity and utter disdain by the medical staff who delivered her. Sally was not placed in her mother's arms, but dumped in a cot at the end of the bed, with the doctor announcing, 'Well, Mrs Johnson, you've got a mongol.' When Sally's mother, Sheila Johnson, asked for some information about Down's syndrome so she could learn more about it she was told, 'Oh no, don't do that, it's all too depressing.' Worse was to follow. Ten days after her birth, the Johnsons had to listen to their then GP advising them that Sally would be 'the village idiot, walking down the street, making hideous sounds, drooling and dribbling. Get rid of that child.' I suppose it was a bedside manner of sorts. . .

Fortunately Sheila, a primary school teacher, ignored her doctor and other health professionals, and was determined to take her daughter home, and for her and her husband to do the best they could for Sally. She battled with the local primary school for it to accept Sally, and then for nearly three years with the education authority, to obtain a place for her at a special school where she knew Sally would be stimulated and achieve her full potential.

Sally was born with an undiagnosed and ultimately fatal heart and lung condition which could have been reversed if the medics had been in the least bit interested in her. Allie and I loved her impressionistic watercolours, which were lucid, full of light and beauty. Sally painted every day and sold more than 2,500 paintings, never keeping a penny for herself and raising thousands of pounds for charity. She worked tirelessly as a volunteer, achieved a gateway Gold Award, wrote poetry and was an avid reader. In her ridiculously short life (she passed away in 2000 at the age of 25), Sally's contribution was more than most of us can ever hope for. 'To be happy, and make others happy' was Sally's credo. Those who met her were touched by her spirit, courage and intelligence; those who didn't know her personally were inspired by her art. I feel extremely privileged to have known Sally, albeit briefly. A paediatrician once told Sheila that Sally would probably grow up to be 'a reasonable cabbage'. Long after this nameless doctor has been forgotten, Sally will long be remembered.

Rachel Heller, born in 1973, is a woman who has made an extraordinary impact on the art world. She produces striking portraits in a style that is clearly personal, and with spontaneity and a lack of inhibition major components in her drawings and etchings, the sense of movement is remarkable. 'The observation is acute and intimate, the execution raw and economic,' the artist Maggi Hambling CBE has said of Rachel's work. 'For me, the work reveals human truth in an eye-opening way.'

Rachel had found it difficult to express herself verbally but, influenced by her family's artistic background – her mother is the gallery owner Angela Flowers and her late father, Robert Heller, an author and management consultant – she soon found within her art a compelling means of self-expression. She started to draw at a very early age and, following an invitation from the Byam School of Art, began to attend life classes on Saturday mornings. Her first show soon followed, and her work has since appeared in several open exhibitions, most notably at the Royal Academy's 2004 Summer Exhibition, and in 2006 she won the Sir Hugh Casson Prize for drawing.

In 2008 Rachel moved out of London to Oxfordshire, and has since been preoccupied with the countryside: her landscapes are portrayed with a similarly expressive tonal range and variety of gestural marks, vigorously applied in pastel. Still-life works on paper, produced between 2001 and 2016, are 'quietly domestic and delicate, with muted tones and hard edges softened by deliberate smudging.'

Art And Soul

It's true to say that the colourfully named Lester Magoogan has a somewhat unique perspective on life. He is, quite simply, a force of nature: his billing matter – if an artist might describe their publicity in music-hall terms, and Lester certainly should – states that 'anyone who has met Lester will never forget the experience!' We have been to one of his shows, a travelling exhibition, entitled 'Lester's World', at which Lester has been present, and he is quite a presence. He produces simple, acutely observed but evocative line drawings, with an essentially abstract approach, and has a wonderfully vivid, surreal sense of humour. His inspiration ranges from TV soaps to gardening, and has been described as 'seeing a seed grow into the plant similar to the start of his art to the finished project.' The late George Melly was an aficionado: 'Lester has all the spontaneity of Miro and Dubuffet but, having no training, there is an immediacy that many great artists have sought within themselves, but few achieve.'

Lester Magoogan is a member of an arts collective known as Heart & Sold, set up to promote artists, photographers and film makers with Down's syndrome, and provide them with a platform where they can develop their art and sell their work. Its director and founder, Suzie Moffat, discovered that there were artists all over the world with Down's syndrome, and was determined that their work should be more widely celebrated, and to 'promote the idea that art is from the heart and has nothing to do with the condition.'

In a recent programme on Radio 4, *The Little Chinese Maiden*, the biographer and poet Grevel Lindop opined that William Wordsworth may well have had a daughter with Down's syndrome. Born in 1808, slow to walk and speak, Catherine was described as a loveable and delightful child with a sweet nature, and was said by William's sister Dorothy to 'have a wonderful sense of humour and something irresistibly comic in her face and movements.' Catherine was especially dear to her father, and used to keep him company in his study while he wrote. The poet referred to her as 'my little Chinese maiden'.

Catherine was small in stature, slower to acquire skills and mobility, and may have had a heart condition. A miniature, painted when Catherine was three, portrays her as having a round face, and the shape of her forehead suggests she had some of the characteristics of a child with Down's. This was over 50 years before John Langdon Down recognised the syndrome, and so Catherine was never labelled, but the clinching description was that she endeared herself to everyone and had a profound effect on those she met and those who loved her!

Wordsworth, who ironically had already penned a sympathetic poem, 'The Idiot Boy', ten years before Catherine was born, wrote two poems about Catherine. The first was 'Characteristics of a Child Three Years Old'.

> Loving she is, and tractable, though wild;
> And Innocence hath privilege in her
> To dignify arch looks and laughing eyes;
> And feats of cunning; and the pretty round
> Of trespasses, affected to provoke
> Mock-chastisement and partnership in play.
> And, as a faggot sparkles on the hearth,
> Not less if unattended and alone
> Than when both young and old sit gathered round
> And take delight in its activity;
> Even so this happy Creature of herself
> Is all-sufficient, solitude to her
> Is blithe society, who fills the air

With gladness and involuntary songs.
Light are her sallies as the tripping fawn's
Forth-startled from the fern where she lay couched;
Unthought-of, unexpected, as the stir
Of the soft breeze ruffling the meadow-flowers,
Or from before it chasing wantonly
The many-coloured images impressed
Upon the bosom of a placid lake.

Catherine died at the age of four in 1812 of unknown causes, although it is thought she had heart problems. Her parents were devastated, and their tragedy was compounded when they lost a second child, Thomas, the very same year. William's sonnet, 'Surprised by Joy', was written soon after, and was thought to have referred to Catherine.

Surprised by joy – impatient as the Wind
I turned to share the transport – Oh! with whom
But Thee, long buried in the silent tomb,
That spot which no vicissitude can find?
Love, faithful love, recalled thee to my mind
But how could I forget thee? Through what power,
Even for the least division of an hour,
Have I been so beguiled as to be blind
To my most grievous loss?
That thought's return was the worst pang that sorrow
ever bore,
Save one, one only, when I stood forlorn,
Knowing my heart's best treasure was no more;
That neither present time, nor years unborn
Could to my sight that heavenly face restore.

A Major Adjustment

A friend of the family, Thomas De Quincey, the essayist and author of *Confessions of an English Opium-Eater*, loved Catherine, and was so heartbroken that he claimed to have slept out on her grave in Grasmere churchyard for six weeks in 'passionate grief'. According to Grevel Lindop, 'it was probably depression following her death that tipped him into full-blown opium addiction.' Children with Down's syndrome do indeed have quite an effect on those they meet...

Acting is another art form which provides people with Down's syndrome with the opportunity to exhibit their talent. Before the millennium characters and storylines in film and television involving Down's syndrome actors were few and far between, but in the last 15 years they have been much more prevalent, both in Europe and across the pond.

In recent years a number of British soaps, such as *Brookside* and *Casualty*, have featured storylines using characters with Down's syndrome. Harry Whittaker, the nephew of the new Dr Who, Jodie Whittaker (an ambassador for Mencap), appeared in *Emmerdale* before his death at the age of just three. In *Coronation Street* the character of Alex Warner has been played by the very talented Liam Bairstow since 2015.

When in 2006 BBC executives decided to introduce a baby with DS into *EastEnders*, copies of *A Minor Adjustment* were given to various members of the cast for research purposes. Subsequently 'Janet' (Grace) was born to Billy and Honey Mitchell, played by Perry Fenwick and Emma Barton. What has been particularly positive about this initiative is that the BBC didn't just use the story purely for its initial drama and then drop the family after the first traumatic few months: Grace has now been in the show on and off for eleven years. According to her parents, Grace loves acting in *EastEnders* and delights in being the show. In 2016 she was even nominated in the 'Best Young Performance' category for a British Soap Award.

Coincidentally, Perry Fenwick lived around the corner from us, and I would occasionally bump into him at our local. Perry met Sarah on several occasions and couldn't have been kinder or more generous to her. For her part she was thrilled to hang out with one of her soap heroes. In fact, Perry and Emma Barton became so embroiled in the Down's syndrome world that they both became patrons of the DSA.

The very popular drama *Call the Midwife*, which is set in the late 1950s and early 1960s, featured an episode in which Reggie, a young man with DS played by Daniel Laurie, loses his parents, leaving him with nowhere to live. The only option is to be moved to a mental asylum, which at the time, as we have already seen, was the case for many with learning disabilities. Also in the cast for that episode was the ex-*EastEnders* actor Cliff Parisi. 'I was around at the time,' recalls Cliff, 'and in the sixties people with Down's were tucked away, but the sister of one of my best friends had Down's and she lived at home, and her mother died, so this story's close to my heart.' Cliff obviously enjoyed working with Daniel: 'We kept singing Cockney songs on set, but he's much more professional than me! He was a delight to work with, and knows exactly what he's doing, so we had a real giggle.'

Sarah Gordy, an actress with Down's syndrome, has also appeared in *Call the Midwife*, as well as *Upstairs, Downstairs*, and more recently in *Strike,* where she gave a touching performance of a woman with severe learning disabilities. In a 2016 interview she was asked, if she could play anyone, who would it be? 'I would like to play a woman where the fact that I have Down's syndrome is part of my character, like my green eyes,' Sarah replied, 'but Down's syndrome is not the story. We do not live in Down's

Syndrome Land, we live, work and play in the same world as everybody else.'

On his website, Otto Baxter, 30, describes himself as 'actor, performer, entertainer extraordinaire'. He has now added 'director' to his repertoire. Otto is all these things and more. Bright, humorous and extrovert, he has featured in several documentaries, and starred in a number of short independent films, including *Two in a Million*, in which a young couple with Down's syndrome face the uncertainties of parenthood. He was also in a short film called *Samuel*, which was shortlisted for the 2016 BAFTA Best British Short Film. For his role in *Ups & Downs* Otto won Best Actor at the Cannes 'Festival Entr'2 Marches' in 2014. As if this wasn't enough, he is currently filming and starring in a musical based on his life which he has written and directed!

It is impossible to write about Otto without describing his family and his remarkable mother. Otto was adopted by Lucy Baxter, who has devoted her life to her four sons, all of whom are adopted and all of whom have Down's syndrome.

Lucy first became involved in the world of learning disability when, at the age of 17 and studying art in Surrey, she worked as volunteer at the Royal Earlswood Hospital, where John Langdon began his medical career, and found herself horrified at the conditions there to which adults and children were subjected. The young 'patients', she discovered, were segregated utterly from the outside world, locked away in a Gothic institution where they might spend their entire lives. Denied personal belongings, toys and books, they even had to share clothes from a communal wardrobe.

> I was expecting people who would all be the same and would just be 'vegetables' – a term that people then

used. But they weren't. They were all much more individual than the rest of us, and were just so deprived – socially, culturally, and materially. Society had let them down and I was a part of that society.

Angered by what she refers to as the 'apartheid of the learning disabled', and frustrated by the lack of change she could achieve at Earlswood, Lucy was determined to make a difference. She therefore decided to apply to adopt a young boy with Down's syndrome. James, now 36, came to live with Lucy when he was five years old. Within a short time, Lucy realised that, apart from Down's syndrome, James was also autistic.

When he was aged seven, Lucy applied to adopt Otto, whose natural parents had been undecided about keeping him, meaning he had remained in foster care until the age of five months. Titus, the third of the Baxter dynasty, is now aged 22, and Lucy's latest addition to the family is Rafi, 14.

Throughout her life Lucy has challenged deeply ingrained prejudices, but hers is not a dogmatic position. She is doing this for her four sons, who she feels should be treated as equal members of society, and afforded the same rights. Lucy wants them all to be independent, and established in employment, friendships and relationships.

The A Word is a BBC TV drama series that centres on a family with a son with autism, but also features a character with Down's, played by the actor Leon Harrop. One of the stars of the show, Christopher Eccleston, described Leon in the *Big Issue* as a 'proper actor, technically brilliant actor. The idea of *The A Word* is to push the door open more and more. It is about visibility and inclusiveness. And then . . . I'm going to become Leon's agent and take over the world and make a lot of money.'

A Major Adjustment

Although these days there are more roles for actors with Down's syndrome, it remains the case that storylines involving characters with Down's tend to be somewhat formulaic – usually involving the death of an ageing relative, and a sympathetic, dependent person with DS who cannot cope on their own and needs a placement or looking after. There are exceptions, of course. The sitcoms *Curb Your Enthusiasm* and *The Inbetweeners* have managed to avoid stereotypes with edgy, funny storylines that involved revenge being wreaked by characters with DS. (I'm a sucker for revenge tales.) Indeed, Larry David, the creator of *Curb* and *Seinfeld*, has a long and distinguished history of creating characters with disabilities who are neither victims nor heroes.

The same cannot be said for Ricky Gervais, whose comedy series *Derek* received much criticism for its cruel portrayal of a man with a learning disability. His use of the word 'mong,' and his posting of pictures of himself making stupid faces to accompany his tweets, didn't endear himself to many people. Still . . . he loves elephants.

A number of American television shows have featured actors with Down's syndrome, and perhaps none more poignantly and successfully than the extraordinarily successful musical vehicle, and one of Sarah's favourite shows, *Glee*. The character of Lauren Potter (Becky Jackson), who has Down's syndrome, is an acid-tongued cheerleader and sidekick to the demonic Sue Sylvester (Jane Lynch). Their unusual friendship is made all the more surprising by Sylvester's vicious nature – but it is later revealed that Sylvester has a sister, Jean, who also has Down's, and she is thus drawn to Lauren. The episode which features Jean's funeral, in which the cast sing the classic *Willy Wonka* tune 'Pure Imagination', is indeed manipulative, but incredibly powerful and emotional.

Adults with learning disabilities feature in several 'reality TV' series. *Born This Way*, an Emmy-winning American television series set in Los Angeles and broadcast in the UK on the Lifetime channel, follows the aspirations, achievements and relationships of seven friends with Down's syndrome. With its unofficial strapline of 'Don't Limit Me', the show has now completed its third series, and has attracted millions of viewers worldwide. Try to think of *Made in Chelsea*, but with real people that you care about, depth of character, charming personalities, important events, meaningful romances, life-changing lessons, inspirational episodes and doting parents. Both entertaining and touching, the show is a triumph. Actually, forget I mentioned *Made in Chelsea*.

Despite its unfortunate title, clearly coined to attract viewers, Channel 4's *The Undateables* is a sympathetically made programme endeavouring to match adults with disabilities, including learning difficulties. The show's treatment of disability has been accused of insensitivity, and its particular mingling of diversity and entertainment as manipulative or even exploitative, but for me the series, in facilitating the participants in their quest for romance and love, does, like its contributors, have its heart in the right place. I also like it that the programme's voice-over commentary is spoken by Sally Phillips, a mover and shaker in the DS world, and if she doesn't approve of any of the text in the script she is given, she will re-word it.

Another award-winning documentary starred Britain's first punk band featuring disabled musicians, who were described by the *Sunday Times* in 2009 as 'possibly the most important punk band touring today.' Referring to themselves as 'Lewes's answer to the Ramones', the members of Heavy Load met at Southdown Housing Association, a non-profit assisted-living community for people with learning difficulties and mental health issues, and were a mix of service users and staff.

A Major Adjustment

Three of the band had some kind of disability: drummer Michael White had Down's syndrome, singer Simon Barker and guitarist Jimmy Nichols learning difficulties, and the film, *Heavy Load: A Film About Happiness*, followed the perpetually chaotic band for two turbulent years. The *Guardian's* music critic, Alexis Petridis, met them in 2008 and reported that the band had three gigs booked over that weekend, but weren't that bothered about rehearsing:

> They play two songs: a cover of Kylie Minogue's 'Can't Get You Out of My Head' that in Heavy Load's hands sounds catastrophic, liking chucking-out time at a particularly rowdy pub, and one of their own called 'We Love George Michael', a hearty thumbs-up for the former Wham! frontman's sexual preferences: 'We love George Michael,' bellow Barker and Williams, more or less in unison, 'because he's gay at weekends and gay in the week.'

Guitarist Mick Williams recalled that the last time drummer Michael White went into a Portaloo before a gig, the band couldn't get him out – although I reckon that probably reflects on the fact that he is a drummer, not because of his Down's. He also mentioned that 'we don't rehearse much because it destroys our spontaneity,' before adding, 'Our music has neither improved nor deteriorated in the last 12 years.'

Heavy Load were together for 15 years, from 1997 to 2012, and during that time performed at hundreds of gigs, playing regularly at disability night clubs and events up and down the country. As they got better known they appeared at two Glastonbury Festivals, and also in New York, Berlin and Copenhagen. They did a few gigs with Sham 69, and once supported the Blockheads.

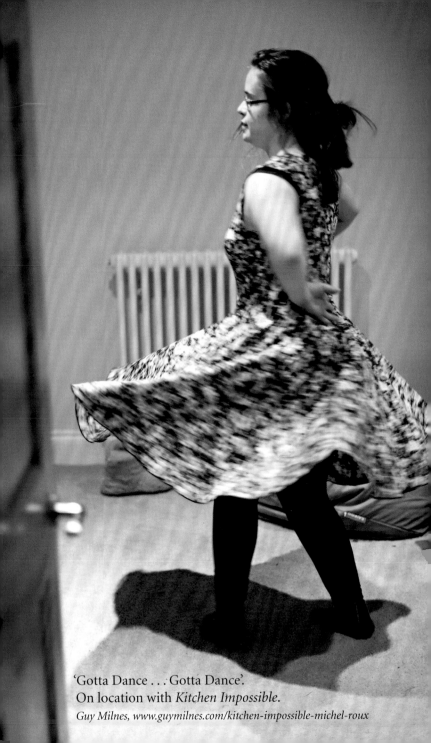

'Gotta Dance . . . Gotta Dance'.
On location with *Kitchen Impossible*.
Guy Milnes, www.guymilnes.com/kitchen-impossible-michel-roux

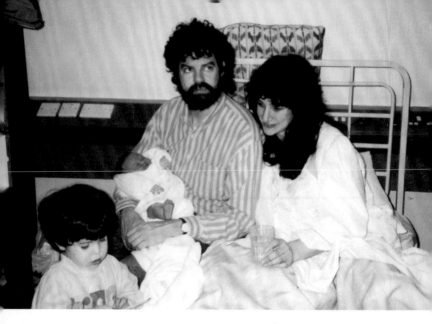

'A little Buddha.' A few hours after Sarah's birth and before 'the icy grip'.

below left: Beach baby. Walberswick, Suffolk.
below right: A Loving Adjustment. *Mark Bernkopf*

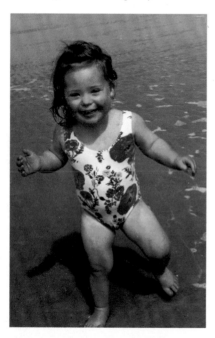

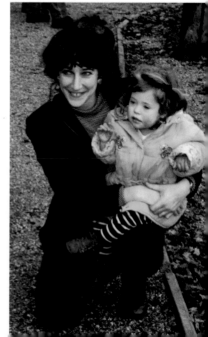

Sarah, Andy and Eric Merriman, junior and senior scribes, *Minor Adjustment*. *BBC/Chris Capstick*

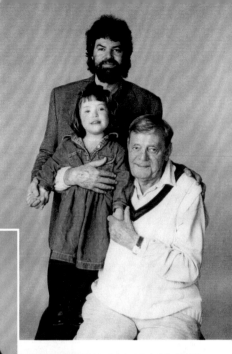

The cast of *Minor Adjustment*: Peter Davison, Clare Russell, Sarah Merriman and Samantha Bond. One of them wasn't potty-trained. *BBC/Chris Capstick*

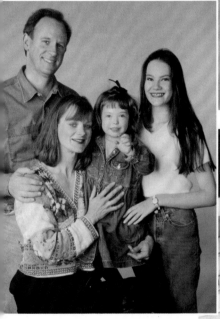

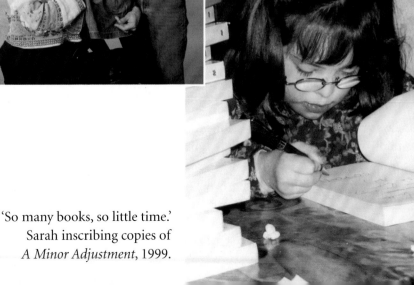

'So many books, so little time.' Sarah inscribing copies of *A Minor Adjustment*, 1999.

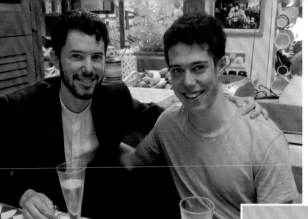

Daniel and Joel, brothers in arms.

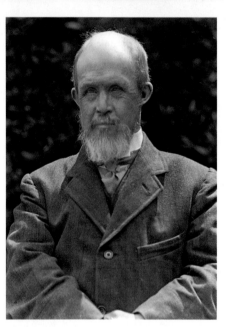

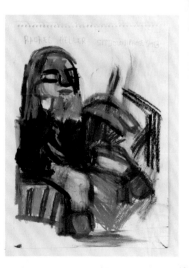

Un-named gentleman in the early days of Normansfield. 'Mongoloid idiot' or 'dignified gentleman'?

above right: A quick sketch by Allie.

right: 'Sit Down Prose', 2013.

© Rachel Heller 2013. *Courtesy of Flowers Gallery London and New York*

The Merrimans with Kevin Kilbane at the Danny Mardell tournament, Upton Park, 2007.

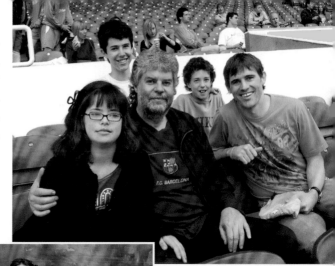

left: 'Girls with attitude'. Left to right: Ophir, Sarah and India.

Fiona Yaron-Field, www.fionayaronfield.co.uk

'Ev'ry Time We Say Goodbye'. Leaving Sarah for the first time at Foxes Academy.

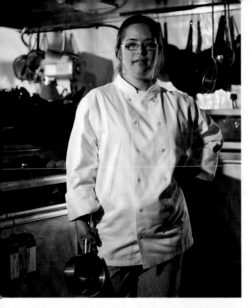

left: Sarah in her 'whites' during the filming of *Kitchen Impossible.*
Hal Shinnie, www.halshinnie.com

below: They'll always have Paris. *Kitchen Impossible* participants and Roux family members. *Guy Milnes*

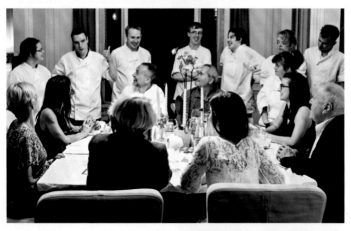

With two of her heroes: Sarah, boyfriend Leon and Michel Roux Jr.
Blake Ezra Photography

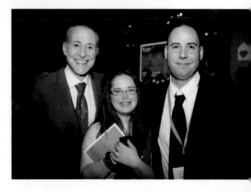

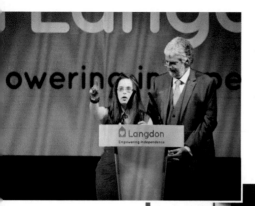

Sarah in full flow at the Langdon charity dinner, Wembley. The author could barely get a word in.
Blake Ezra Photography

right: The customer is king: Sarah at work at the Thistle Hotel Brasserie. *Clare Walsh*

below: A happy return to Foxes.

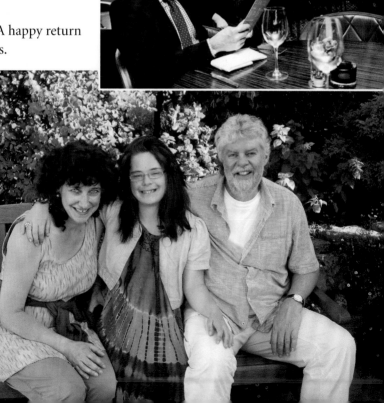

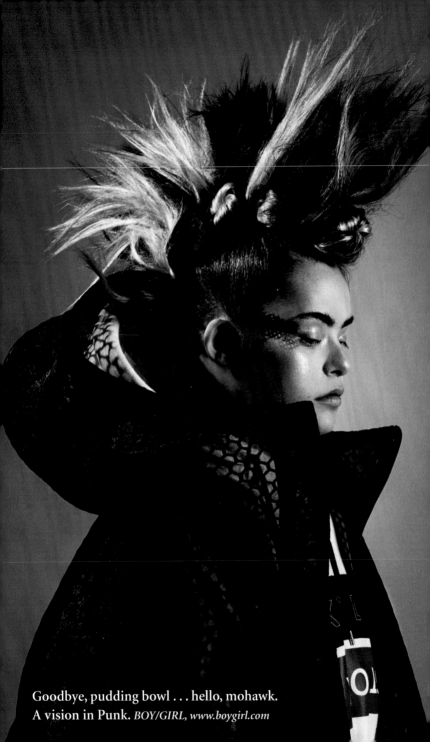

Goodbye, pudding bowl . . . hello, mohawk.
A vision in Punk. *BOY/GIRL, www.boygirl.com*

Art And Soul

Tragically, frontman Simon Barker died in August 2017, and the band held an open-night karaoke event to find a new singer should the band ever reform. Simon, along with support worker and fellow band member Paul Richards, had been one of the founders of Stay Up Late, a charity set up to allow support workers to be given flexible rotas so they could accompany adults with learning disabilities to gigs and social events – something the rest of us take for granted. While my son Daniel was at Sheffield University he volunteered for something similar called Clubbing Crew.

A number of actors with Down's first trod the boards with dance and theatre companies. Kaleidoscope Theatre was founded as the first company of its kind in 1980. Its shows are created entirely in-house, and performed by its actors, of all ages and from varied walks of life, with little money but with a passion for their story. Kaleidoscope has performed in many venues over the years, and at least a dozen times at the Edinburgh Fringe. The company has also provided extras and minor parts for a number of mainstream films.

Blue Apple Theatre provides 'high-quality, ambitious theatre and dance opportunities to people with disabilities, with no disabling through low expectation.' The company celebrated its tenth anniversary with a tour of *Hamlet* and a performance at Shakespeare's Globe, which was filmed for a BBC documentary, *Growing Up Down's*, which won the TV Creativity Diversity award for best new programme and was nominated for an international Emmy.

A member of the Blue Apple company, Tommy Jessop, also a talented dancer, has appeared in *Casualty*, *Holby City* and a BBC television film, *Coming Down the Mountain*, in which his character was initially the target of a murderous plot by his brother – a nice change, I have to say, from the usual plotlines.

A Major Adjustment

He has recently undertaken another interesting role, of a boxer, in a short film, *Fighter*, shown at the 2017 London Film festival, for which he has received rave reviews.

Chicken Shed is a nationally well-known integrated theatre company which provides training, workshops and innovative productions that include children and adults with learning difficulties. Sarah participated in a couple of its Christmas productions, in one camouflaged as a tree. Friends who went to see it didn't realise she had actually been on stage. The other role, as a scallop, didn't further her theatrical career, although if ever there is a West End production of *The Little Mermaid* she would stand a fighting chance.

It was actually Chicken Shed's local counterpart, Haringey Shed, in which Sarah was more involved. Based in Tottenham, Haringey Shed genuinely reflects the rich diversity of the community, and is a truly inclusive theatre company offering professional performing-arts opportunities to children and young people aged 7–16. There are no auditions: everyone is welcome regardless of ability, and no child is excluded because of inability to pay fees.

Sarah initially attended a mentoring group on Saturday mornings when she was in her teens. Through storytelling and role play, she was given the opportunity to learn and pass on skills, which provided her with an added sense of responsibility and self-confidence.

Over the years, we have attended several performances, and never failed to marvel at the extraordinary energy, enthusiasm, talent and joy of the participants and the obvious dedication of the helpers. (Apart from employing a small number of staff, who are truly dedicated and often work far beyond the call of duty, Haringey Shed depend on over 50 volunteers from the local community.)

The company's activities include theatre, music, dance and outreach programmes, involving over 2,000 children and young people each year, many of whom have never had access to the performing arts. There is also outreach work in schools, work experience and volunteering opportunities for young people with special needs. Much of the work is devised by the young people themselves. A weekly theatre group always ends in a musical production, and Sarah participated in an incredibly imaginative production of *Romeo and Juliet* transposed to competing supermarkets. The play was devised from scratch by the participants themselves, who in just five days created a highly original and uplifting production with original music.

It wasn't until 1996 that a major cinematic work featured a character with Down's syndrome, when a Belgian actor, Pascal Duquenne, co-starred in *The Eighth Day* and shared the Best Actor prize at the Cannes Film Festival with his co-star Daniel Auteuil. Since then, however, characters with Down's have had much more of a presence.

According to Alison Peebles, the director of *Afterlife* (2003), all the cast and crew had personal associations with Down's or special needs, or at least an empathetic sensitivity, which clearly influenced the project. The film follows an ambitious journalist who learns that his mother is dying, leaving him to assume responsibility for his disabled sister Roberta, portrayed by debutante Paula Sage. A touching relationship develops between the siblings, forcing Roberta's brother to reassess his life. *Afterlife* is also realistic, because Andrea Gibb's script was inspired by her own sister, Sharon, who has Down's. Paula manages both drama and humour in equal measures, and is a natural performer.

Any Day Now (2012) is a terrific film, set in the late 1970s and inspired by a true story, and relates a tale of love, difference and acceptance. Marco (Isaac Leyva), a teenager with Down's syndrome, has been abandoned by his addicted, prostitute mother. He is taken in by a struggling drag queen, Rudy, played by the marvellous Alan Cumming, who enlists his partner Paul (Garret Dillahunt) in the battle to give Rudy a secure and loving home. Marco finds in them the family he's never had, but when their alternative living arrangements are discovered by the authorities, Rudy and Paul are denied the opportunity to adopt the child they have come to love as their own. The trio discover that the courts are against gay adoptive parents and the couple must fight to retain custody of Marco, despite the fact that the alternative could be an institution. Both the gay men and Marco are 'outsiders', kept out of the mainstream by prejudice and ignorance.

Although *My Feral Heart* (2016) explored a familiar theme, of a young man with Down's syndrome being placed in an institution following a family bereavement, it combined the principal plotline with a dash of magical realism, and was released to critical acclaim. The film's lead, Steven Brandon, won the Best Actor award at the National Film Awards for an extraordinary performance.

A double BAFTA winner in 2015 was the BBC film *Marvellous*, which charts the life and true story of Neil Baldwin, a man with a learning disability, in his various guises as professional clown, student mentor and Stoke City kit man! As Baldwin, Toby Jones gave a wonderfully understated performance in a drama that helped bring to a wider audience the challenges of people with learning disabilities. It wasn't just Neil Baldwin himself who has benefited from being accepted into mainstream life, the film showed: he has enriched the lives of people around him – in the 1990s, when Neil became a kit man for Stoke City, the club's manager Lou Macari described him as 'the best signing I ever made.' It wasn't something done out of pity or sympathy: Neil brought his own unique personality to the job – although he had originally applied to be the manager. 'I always wanted to be happy,' says Neil in the film, 'so I decided to be.' It's as simple as that. With a welcoming and supportive community, people with learning disabilities can achieve this modest goal . . . and so much more.

It is interesting to note that one in five people has some form of disability, but this 20 per cent of the population accounts for just over one per cent of those appearing on television. In the US, 95 per cent of television characters are played by non-disabled actors.

Someone once said, 'We should consider every day lost on which we have not danced at least once.' It was either Friedrich Nietzsche or Fred Astaire, I forget which, but whoever it was, the sentiment captures the freedom of spirit and ability to express oneself that dance can bring to everyone's life: a feeling of liberation and articulacy of movement all the greater, moreover, when speech might prove difficult. There are a number of inclusive dance companies that provide just such an opportunity for children and adults with learning difficulties.

Candoco is a professional dance company specialising in the integration of disabled and non-disabled artists, which developed out of integrated workshops at London's Aspire Centre for Spinal Injury, and quickly grew into the first company of its kind in the UK. However, the original artistic director Celeste Dandeker's priority was that Candoco should be run, and judged, as a dance company, not a therapeutic project. This vision was reflected in her ambitious commissioning strategy, catapulting it into the mainstream dance world from the very beginning. Since then Candoco has performed across the globe, having visited over 25 countries since 2002, and performed at venues such as the Bird's Nest in Beijing and the Olympic Stadium in London, performing at the handover ceremonies in

2008 and returning, alongside Coldplay, at the Paralympics' closing in 2012.

Sarah's friend Ophir has been a member of Candoco for nine years, and has nothing but praise for the company.

> I feel free when I dance. I love the creative choreography, and I like how they help me think and learn about dance. My dance teachers and dance friends accept me for who I am and my abilities to dance.
>
> It is amazing to perform out in the world. We have been to many places, and I have also been helping to lead the Candoco movement workshop at Tate Britain. In Bestival [a boutique music festival in Dorset] I shared a tent with a lovely buddy for two nights. It was the first time I was away from home, on my own. There I loved performing on stage, and having a lot of fun with my dance friends.
>
> *Traces of War* was a different experience. We were working with war veterans and students from King's College. We all created a dance which was based around 'war', inspired by meeting the artists for a chat and looking at the art work. It was very challenging. At the end of an intensive week, we all performed the dance we have created in the gallery space of Somerset House.

Ophir's younger sister Noa is also involved with the company.

> I've come to learn more about the importance of inclusive dance. In my opinion, Candoco isn't just providing opportunities for people with disabilities:

it's expanding views around dance. Dance can be a world of uniformity and rigidity, which Candoco consistently challenges. They don't see difference as something to overcome, rather they see it as an asset, a way to expand dance beyond the traditional ideas. The company is filled with creative, talented people. Sometimes with inclusive dance there's a tendency for the piece to become a sympathy act, but in Candoco the quality of dance is never compromised. It is art, and inclusion only furthers this, not hinders it.

The company has had a hugely positive and significant effect on the lives of me and my sister. I have watched my sister grow in confidence, and discover somewhere she can truly express her passion in a compassionate environment that truly pushes. For me, what started as an after-school activity has developed into discovering a true love and interest for dance.

It is not always easy. There are times where I struggle to find a balance between looking after someone else, and looking after myself. However, when these challenges arise they always seem to result in me discovering something new and progressing. I have found Candoco the most supportive place in encouraging creativity.

Andrew Self is a breathtakingly graceful and elegant performer who dances with Cando2, Candoco's youth company. He has recently freestyled (choreographed) and performed in his debut music video, and has even done some dance busking outside the London Palladium! Currently he is a second-year day student at the Orpheus Centre, a further education college for young disabled people with a passion for the performing arts.

'I can see such a difference in his first shows, when he was quite hesitant,' comments his mother, Donna. 'Now he relishes being on stage, and nothing fazes him – he is joy personified! Dancing has increased Andrew's confidence greatly because he knows it is something he excels at – he loves entertaining, and seeing people enjoy his performances.' In Andrew's own words, 'Dancing makes me feel happy and ecstatic.' He also attends weekly classes with StopGap, a Farnham-based dance company under the artistic direction of Lucy Bennett, that encourages disabled and non-disabled artists to collaborate. The actors Tommy Jessop and Sarah Gordy also dance with StopGap.

I am aware that I've only referred to theatre and dance companies with which Sarah has been involved, or with which we have personal links. I realise there are other arts organisations all over the UK, and many talented performers who also deserve a mention. As that old music-hall comedian and part-time Roman emperor Marcus Aurelius once remarked, 'Remember this, that there is a proper value and proportion to be observed in the performance of every act.'

9

FURTHER PATERFAMILIAS TERRITORY

Happy father's day I hope you have fulfilled day with happiness and joy your always be my partner in crime and being my best dad 4 ever since24 years best years of my life I wish I was with you today could I speak to you soon I love you you're my best dad I miss you AlwAys when I'm not around you because we have dad and daughter bonding time. I missed it ok i love you loads

A text from Sarah, Father's Day (19 June 2016)

Within a week of Sarah's birth, we received a letter that was to have a profound effect on our ability to come to terms with our situation. Ken Hixon is a screenwriter based in Hollywood and, although we had never met, we shared a mutual friend in Sarah's godfather. Paul Kelly had telephoned Ken and his wife Melanie immediately with our news.

A Major Adjustment

Dear Ally and Andrew,

My name is Ken Hixon, I am the father of Lilian Hixon, who happens to be one of my most noteworthy accomplishments. Lily is eight years old, a girl of extraordinary will, affection, humour and beauty, and lower on the list with her other vital statistics would be the notation 'Down syndrome'.

Not that it isn't obvious that Lily has Down syndrome, indeed she has all the characteristics, but what strikes people first and foremost about Lily is her joyful and amazing personality. I'm certain my bias is quite blatant by now. But beyond my bond to her as father to child, as a somewhat eccentric person myself, and married to a woman of distinct individuality, what draws me so tightly to Lily is her utter uniqueness. She is one of the most original people I've ever met. She is fearless, but astutely sensitive. She is clumsy, but innately poised. She is an anarchist with a Zen-like zeal for ritual and routine. I think the word is contradictions. An apt word for Lily and for many of the feelings and experiences her mother and I have had.

To say that giving birth to a child with Down Syndrome was a painful shock is, as you already know, a sublime understatement. But graced as we were by the affections of our friends and family, the level-headed advice of our paediatrician, and our own stamina and love for each other, my wife Melanie and I rose, somewhat wobbly, to the challenge at hand.

Not without pain nor tears, not without insecurities and confusion. But simply. The best advice we received early on was just to take our new baby home and enjoy her. That there is ample time to become experts on mental retardation. We learned the wisdom of this immediately. We just took a breath and found that Lily's needs were no more complex than any other infant's – she needed to be fed, bathed, changed, hugged, kissed, held, and made funny faces at. In fact, after just a few months I decided that if Lily is retarded then I must be retarded as well, because she made perfect sense to me.

Her so-called 'slow' development was just my speed. In fact after the birth of our son, Sam, we labelled him 'severely normal'. Indeed, it would be a toss-up determining which child has placed the most demands on us as parents. Of course I don't mean to brush aside the enormous amount of energy and effort to meet the needs of a child with Down Syndrome. And I certainly do not wish to infer that I have no concern for the social 'slings and arrows' Lilian will suffer in this oh-so-perfect world. I do worry. I do get depressed. I am anxious at times, but most of the time, the overwhelming majority of the time, I am just in love with Lily.

I would be lost without her.

All my best,
Ken Hixon

A Major Adjustment

Allie and I were both incredibly moved by the letter – not just the beautifully written content, but by the efficiency with which the network had begun to spread the news and the speed with which Ken had composed and posted this missive. Lily, a complete stranger 6,000 miles away, had entered our lives in the same way that our own daughter had done a few days earlier. And this, of course, was before the days of email, when we might have received this extraordinary missive even sooner.

Was it really possible that Sarah could achieve what Lily had achieved in only eight years? Could Sarah become a similar character – an individual, full of potential and with her own unique personality?

It also touched us that this couple – unknown to us until this letter – had faced the very same situation eight years previously, and had survived the ordeal. The family seemed to be so very different from the image I kept thinking of – a family burdened by the addition of a disabled child, struggling from one crisis to the next, and unable to lead a 'normal' life. They were optimistic about the future, but not mindlessly impervious to the troubles that would arise from time to time.

And as for Lily . . . well, we just loved her already. Despite the fact that we had never met her, we were completely smitten. Maybe we could fall in love with our own daughter sometime in the future? If Ken and Melanie could discover so much love for Lily, then why couldn't we? Here was a dad who would be lost without his daughter.

Allie carried this letter everywhere, and read it constantly for the first month after Sarah's birth. It became a sort of Down's syndrome passport, 'allowing the bearer to pass freely without let or hindrance and to afford the bearer such assistance and protection as may be necessary'. We could venture into unknown territory and unexplored lands with this document, and it would also enable the bearer to discuss the subject of Down's syndrome at any time with any person. The letter would be produced in a flash and thrust upon any friend, acquaintance or member of the public who had unwittingly shown even a passing interest. Supermarket shoppers idly checking the 'Kosher Korner' for a deal on sweet cucumbers or chopped herring, and who paused for a moment to smile at Sarah, would receive a five-minute lecture on special needs and a copy of the letter.

Following Sarah's cardiac scan at the Whittington, she was then referred to an eminent paediatric heart specialist at the Brompton and, instead of handing him the referral letter from Dr Mackinnon, by mistake Allie handed him Ken Hixon's letter. He read it for a couple of minutes, becoming more and more puzzled, until he handed us back the letter and said, 'Lily seems like a nice girl, but what is this to do with me?' I am still convinced that he only realised it wasn't a letter from another doctor because he could read the writing.

Incidentally, Lily, now in her mid-thirties, is happily married to Jonny, a gentle giant who hails from south central Los Angeles. They live semi-independently in Monrovia, a suburb of the city, and tied the knot some years ago in a rather grand wedding. As Ken said at the time, 'Lily doesn't play small venues.' We have stayed in touch with the family, and vist them in Los Angeles whenever we can. As I mentioned previously, Lily and Jonny made cameo appearances in *Born This Way*, dispensing marital advice to a younger couple who had just become engaged.

In the first few days after Sarah was born, and before Allie came home from hospital, I started to make contact with friends about the news. Although at the time it certainly didn't feel that it was helping me to come to terms with the situation, it was in fact a very valuable process. Generally the reactions from people ranged from, 'Jesus Christ, what a nightmare,' to 'So, what's the problem?' and even, 'Sarah will be such a challenge – I'm excited for you both.' I suppose we were grateful for any contact, and I would certainly not be critical of anyone's first responses to such dramatic news. I know that if I had been put on the spot like that, I just wouldn't have had any idea of what to say, or how to say it.

Following her discharge from hospital, Sarah had to be brought back to the Special Care Baby Unit every day to ascertain that her liver was functioning normally. It was agreed that I would take her back to the hospital each morning for a blood test, as Allie certainly didn't want to face the hospital staff, or indeed the rest of the world, and I was happy to take on this job, as I felt at least there was something practical that I could do. I was pleased that I was being useful and taking an active part in the first week of Sarah's life. Apart from protecting Allie and breaking the news to people, I had a role.

Historically, the father's role has been regarded as primarily social and economic, whereas the mother's was essentially bio-logical and nurturing. We now know that this does not have to be the case. Women can do anything that men can do. Likewise, the notion of childcare, which even now remains very much in the female domain need not be so bound by traditional roles. The practicalities of childcare hold no mystique – anyone can cuddle, wash, bathe, dress, undress or feed a baby, change a nappy, and then put him or her to bed. When it comes to parenting, there is little that a man cannot do except be pregnant, give birth to a baby and breastfeed. Even in breastfeeding, some men tried to get in on the act.

Further Paterfamilias Territory

Nearly 30 years ago Allie was doing an analytical counselling course, and we had dinner with a couple of her colleagues and their partners. We had all just become parents for the first time, and inevitably the discussion turned to raising children. Two of the men, precious in the extreme, were bemoaning the fact that they were unable to breastfeed. Biologically bereft, they spoke of the loss they felt, and how this vital bonding process was denied them because they were men.

One of them had discovered a pouch which could be placed around the male pectorals and then filled with milk, so that newborn babies could find succour from their pater. The father could then be part of the breastfeeding process, and be a 'proper' parent. I was utterly appalled, and said something along the lines of, 'Call me Neanderthal, but I would rather stick needles in my eyes than do that.' They were horrified, and looked at Allie with great pity. She had obviously made a terrible mistake in marrying a man who had no wish to breastfeed his firstborn.

In *A Minor Adjustment*, I interviewed a number of fathers, mainly with children under ten years old, about their role, hopes and aspirations, and their feelings about having a child with Down's. In the 1990s, despite the changing nature of the parental roles, there remained a stereotypical expectation of the father. We were still meant to be brave and strong. We had to 'cope' whilst maintaining a sense of calm, and provide the principal source of emotional and practical sustenance. And yet we were also expected to share our feelings, and be honest in our fears and concerns. We were allowed to show our pain. This dichotomy was keenly felt by many fathers, who stated that their main perceived role was to support their partners, wives and families, and to be the ones who 'keep it all together'. Most of the fathers felt that they had to be 'responsible' and 'positive' in the face of adversity, no matter how desperate they were feeling themselves. It is now a little more normal to be 'a stay-at-home dad', but otherwise roles haven't changed that much.

As we've seen, one of the first tasks of the dad after the birth is to contact relatives and friends. When you have had a child with Down's syndrome, the task isn't quite so straightforward, and the fathers I spoke to all found the experience extremely upsetting and very emotional.

One father said he 'told people in an apologetic way, as if I was guilty of some kind of offence'. A number of the dads tried to be upbeat themselves, to make it easier for the recipient of the phone call, and one stated that he was deliberately cheerful in order to reassure everyone else. He wanted them to celebrate the child's birth as usual, and tried to put them at their ease by being positive.

That particular reaction was unusual then, whereas nowadays there exists among some parents a much more positive attitude to having a child with Down's. What is very clear is how the current generation of fathers are much more militant in their opposition to any negative language as used by medical staff at the birth of their child. 'Congratulations!' is now the expected salutation, rather than 'I'm sorry.' When it comes to pre-natal testing, terms like 'risk' of Down's syndrome are not welcome: 'chance' or 'likelihood' is more acceptable. And talking about 'suffering from Down's Syndrome' is strictly non-U.

The fathers' reactions to the birth were a mixture of anxiety, devastation, sadness, disappointment and 'a sense of failure'. Two of their immediate reactions were, 'No matter what he's like, he's gorgeous and he's ours,' and, 'We would love him just the same whatever happens.' The most positive responses came from fathers whose wives had had previous miscarriages or stillbirths, and were relieved that their babies had been born safe and sound. The diagnosis of Down's syndrome was very much a secondary and less important factor in these dads' responses.

One father was traumatised, and wanted his daughter 'to be taken away'. His mind was, swiftly changed, however, by the attitude of his wife, who accepted her newborn baby quickly and unreservedly. 'This immediate bond my wife had with this newborn child has become the most powerful and close relationship I have witnessed in my entire life.'

I've heard of one dad who tried to smother his child, and one who wished he could wave a magic wand and make the Down's syndrome disappear, but my favourite immediate response is exquisite in its simplicity and directness, and has a universal male appeal. This father decided to take up karate, because he wanted to make sure that no one was going to insult his son and get away with it!

After the initial shock, the fathers coped in myriad ways: they found solace in friends and family, faith, and various support groups, and a number read books on the subject to gain information. Whilst their wives and partners were trying to cope with it emotionally, some of the dads were attempting to digest it intellectually.

For some while Allie and I were approached by friends of friends and organisations who wanted advice or simply a chat about Down's. We were of course more than happy to help in any way. When Sarah was about eight, a couple came to see us with their daughter, who was barely a month old. While the child's mother was tearful and emotional, the husband had spent the weeks since the birth of their child researching the subject of Down's in every conceivable way. He already had an answer for everything I tried to discuss with him. In fact, he knew more about

Down's syndrome than I ever would. I didn't know whether to be impressed or disappointed, but hoped that in time he would grow to love her for who she was, rather than seeing her as an academic exercise.

Generally it seemed that the father felt pressure to get on with things as quickly as possible, and immerse himself in the practicalities. 'I did all the washing and ironing – it helped me to find that there was some small domestic routine I could stay in control of when everything else seemed chaotic.' Another father described the first few months as a 'state of siege', having to 'batten down the hatches'.

Work played a large part in this adjustment, as a way of returning to some sort of normality. Of course, some of the fathers had to return to their jobs very quickly after the birth, and one or two felt that their most valuable contribution was that of provider, but it was also clear that they were relieved to use work as a way of escaping the stress at home.

I also found that the main role of the fathers I interviewed was that of propping up their partners, who on the whole took longer to accept what had happened. Many of the fathers took on a very protective role, and said that they felt much more sympathy for their wives. 'I felt sorry for my wife, who so wanted a daughter. Somehow we believed this thing we had brought into the world could never be a daughter. How wrong my daughter has proved us.'

It is the mothers who carry the child through pregnancy, and they who often take on the responsibility for what has happened. Many of the wives felt intensely unhappy, considering themselves 'failures', and felt guilty about having a child with Down's syndrome. The fathers were unable to remove the burden of responsibility from the mother.

Further Paterfamilias Territory

When the child was born, there was general agreement that they had got the sex of the child they had wanted. 'Glad he's a boy, because he's less vulnerable to exploitation and won't get pregnant.' 'We wanted a girl, so we were pleased.' 'We would have more anxieties about a girl. It's easier for a boy to fit in socially and be "one of the lads."' 'I'm pleased that she's a girl – there is a belief that girls are more able.' Of course, there's likely to be a degree of rationalisation in order to accept what has happened. We certainly did this with Sarah, and spoke of how grateful we were that she was the second-born, so that we had some experience of raising a child in ordinary circumstances before she arrived.

Most of the fathers felt that they had experienced some fundamental changes to their outlook on life: the world was definitely felt to be a less benign place, and most of the fathers felt increased feelings of insecurity. One dad described how it had made him more spiritual: he was now more affected by world events, and the experience had put everything into perspective. He felt that his daughter's existence had given him a greater integrity. One father whose job is primarily concerned with communication said that his daughter had helped him to communicate better. She had challenged his preconceptions of aesthetics, and he said he was now much more tolerant when it came to levels of ability and achievement. He spoke of his intense relationship with his daughter, which had resulted in 'unconditional love'. He would never be the same person, he said: 'Only good has come out of the whole experience.'

When I asked the fathers why they thought this had happened to them, most replied it was just 'the luck of the draw', 'the cruelty and capriciousness of fate', 'just the way it is'. In one case it was a matter of 'God's way of trying to get your attention by giving you a slap around the head'. But there was also talk of some 'fault' being involved: a feeling that it was divine retribution for past discrepancies. One man spent months and years desperately trying to find a reason why it had happened, and wondered if he was being punished for doing something wrong. He had lived a fairly charmed life, and now was convinced he was 'paying the price'.

I once had a huge confrontation with an acquaintance who informed me that Sarah's condition was due to 'karma'. He was adamant – and didn't seem to mind telling us quite bluntly – that Sarah had commited some misdemanour, or more likely 'a major wrong', in a previous life, and was now paying the price. In other words, 'you get what you deserve.' I was incensed, but could only summise that he must have graduated from the Miss Agatha Trunchbull Academy of Spiritual Indeterminacy. Anyway, I later discovered that he had left his wife and run off with her money. Goodness knows what she must have done in a previous life to deserve his disappearance, but it must have been something wonderful.

For this book, I've re-interviewed some of the same fathers, and also talked to new dads, to ascertain how the situation has changed in terms of their roles and involvement. How, I wondered, had having a child with DS changed these fathers' views and perceptions of themselves?

> 'She has a unique quality to her life, and has made me a better person. I can learn from her – she is now teaching me how to use my iPad. I'm more patient. I understand a different timeframe, different pace.'

> 'I'm much more stoical than I would have been. I'm not sure I'd have liked the person I would have been without my son.'

'I became an activist and threw myself into the politics of disability rights, and became frustrated with other dads who didn't see my point. I see myself and my wife as advocates when our son can't speak for himself. I haven't always done well, and used to see red if my son had been discriminated against. I'm now more conciliatory.'

'My daughter's Down's syndrome has driven me to provide and work all I can for my family. I'm able to use my occupation to influence my work colleagues about disability.'

'It's opened my eyes to all forms of disability and intolerance.'

'I might be wrong, but I believe I've become a far better human being. Less arrogant, less selfish and far more patient. Having my daughter has changed me without a doubt. She generally has such a lovely outlook on life that it can't help rub off on you. I've learned to be more patient, less stressful. It has also made me more understanding of children and adults with all disabilities, and encouraged me to help and interact with those who have a physical or mental disability.'

'I've learned to confront my own mortality, which is something I would never have done. I'm much more analytical than I ever would have been.'

A Major Adjustment

The breaking of the news that your child has Down's was always problematic, and doctors can never get it completely right – the very nature of the news they are about to impart makes it impossible for them to judge every situation correctly. There is a likelihood that the parents of a child born with a disability will always be dissatisfied with the way they are told. There is no easy way, but it's true that bad practice still exists, and often tactless and insensitive things are said by medical staff who should by now know better. One couple was told, 'She might know your name, walk, talk' and, 'You'll be lucky if she can read MEN or WOMEN on a toilet door.'

One father named their obstetrician 'Dr Doom', because of his gloomy misdemeanour and his declaration that 'We suspect your baby has Down's syndrome.' Looking back, he and his wife wished they hadn't received such a melancholic pronouncement. Although they didn't want an 'over the top' song-and-dance number – 'Hurrah, your daughter has Down's!' – they felt there must be a middle way of breaking the news.

'When my wife was 19 weeks pregnant,' another father told me,

> she received a phone call at work in which the midwife told her the baby was 'affected' by Down's syndrome. It was delivered with an undertone of bad news. When we went back to meet with the consultant a few days later, the conversation was very much geared towards termination, and the assumption was that we would indeed terminate the pregnancy. When we were much further along with the pregnancy (and had firmly decided we were keeping the baby), a consultant told us that, should we change our minds, we would still be able to end the pregnancy at 36 plus weeks. This

was repeated at the end of every consultation, even though we were clearly positive about our choice to continue with the pregnancy.

'Later, during the eight days in hospital that followed, various pieces of the news were broken. A consultant came in and explained "how this could have all been avoided" – not what we wanted to hear, and something we subsequently complained about. My baby daughter's genetic test to confirm the diagnosis was not even discussed with us in person.'

I questioned some of the dads about what they considered to be the most difficult thing about having a child with Down's: the existence of a dual diagnosis – of heart problems, autism or other conditions. Without question, it was the families whose children also suffered from medical problems who experienced the most disruption to their lives. One dad's daughter, aged 15, is on the autistic spectrum, and also suffers from an anxiety disorder. She finds change and new things difficult, and planning and strategies for such events are vital.

The problem of friendships, or lack of them, was universal. The gap between the children with DS and their peers sometimes seemed unbridgeable. It was common that most had no friends beyond the learning-disability community, and could find themselves socially isolated. Differences were highlighted at parties and gatherings when they left 'the bubble of their own home'. 'My son isn't disabled,' one dad told me, 'until he leaves the house.'

One father found it painfully difficult to embrace the 'Down's syndrome part' of his daughter at first, and still finds it tough. She is now in her 20's and is incredibly bright, but this presents its own difficulties, as she 'falls between two worlds'. He wants what's best for her, but is still confused about what is 'the best'? To continue to challenge and motivate her, or let her do the things she wants to do that make her happy? 'If she had her way, she would spend the day watching television and eating crap.'

Another dad was stunned by the depth of negative feelings when his daughter was born, and how he experienced a deep sense of shame. 'I felt that I lacked a basic biological functionality – there was something wrong with my sperm. I'd failed.' Despite how shocked and depressed he felt at his daughter's birth, however, while his wife slept he held his baby all through that first night she was born, and promised her that, whatever happened, he would love her and look after her all her life. He made a promise never to let her down, and is proud that he has done just that. He hated the perception of being defined as the father of a child with a disability and at first raged against everyone and everything, shocked at the prejudices he didn't even knew he possessed. It took him seven years to be able 'to function truthfully in public'. Despite this, it never affected the way he felt about his daughter, and despite his preconceptions he found the capacity to love her.

One father was unequivocal in his feelings about his daughter:

> 'I've loved every minute with my daughter, and if someone came to me with a miracle 'cure' for Down's syndrome next week, I would refuse point-blank. She is who she is, and in some ways having DS has defined her as a person . . . she embraces the fact she has Down's syndrome, and wears it like a badge of honour. I sometimes suggest that maybe I could take part in some of the activities she does at her excellent weekend

group, and her immediate response is, "Don't be silly, Daddy – you haven't got Down's syndrome!"'

Most dads expressed concerns about their children not reaching their full potential: 'He'll never achieve the same as his siblings. He knows that he is different, and doesn't want to be.' Several fathers said they couldn't leave their sons on their own, even though they were teenagers – so a short break, or even a meal out, was problematic. Plans or arrangements always had to be made, and any spontaneity was impossible. One dad was frustrated by society's obsession with testing and quantifying, and the inflexibility of the educational system. He was particularly dissatisfied that school reports state whether a child is working above, below or to expectation. By the very nature of Down's, his daughter is always working below expectation, so they cannot actually show her her school report, because she would get too upset.

There were several 'escapee' stories about their offspring making a break for it, running away or innocently going on journeys to school or see friends without informing their parents of their plans. Several desperate families had to ring the police, and helicopters were even used in various searches. Apart from fears for the safety of their children, some were also concerned about the reaction from the rescuers. When one girl ran away and was found, having decided to make her own way to her school rather than waiting for the school bus, a copper told her mother, 'Don't worry, we won't be taking it any further. You mustn't feel you're a bad mother.'

'My son will sometimes try and leave the house and go walkabout,' one dad told me.

We now keep all the downstairs windows and door double-locked, so he can't escape. The first time he left we didn't realise for a while, and had to call the police. He was eventually found walking down the North Circular Road. The police said it was easy to spot him as he was wearing his pyjamas, a pair of oversized wellington boots and was carrying a backpack.

'When my daughter was five,' recalled another,

we were celebrating my mother-in-law's 70th birthday at a hotel which had other functions going on in other parts of the venue. At one stage we couldn't find her – we all thought she was with somebody else – and the sinking panic set in. We set off in all directions looking for her, thinking she may have wandered upstairs or outside. Eventually my wife found her dancing in the middle of the dance floor at a wedding that was also taking place in the venue. There was a crowd around her clapping and cheering!! Not sure where they thought their little entertainer had come from, but we were very relieved to find her safe and sound.

Nearly every father reported that having a child with Down's syndrome had strengthened the relationship with their partners, and created an even closer bond with other family members. Despite the extra stress, pressure and general fatigue, they felt closer to their partner. This actually concurs with a number of studies which show that the level of marital disharmony and the rate of separation and divorce are no higher among parents who have a child with Down's syndrome. The acceptance from extended family members was imperative from birth, and continuing support and love throughout couldn't have been more valuable.

Siblings, naturally, played an integral role within the family, and most were influenced positively by having a brother or sister with a disability. One teenager with a sibling with Down's made a YouTube video about the derogatory use of the word 'retard', and five of his schoolfriends said they would never use the 'R' word again. His girlfriend also had to pass the test of spending time with his brother, and he made it quite clear to her that if she hadn't accepted and welcomed his brother, she wouldn't have been his girlfriend for very long!

Apart from being fiercely loyal and protective, the siblings were so much more empathetic, aware of disability than their peers, and many had volunteered with groups for the learning-disabled. Some were even planning careers in the 'caring professions'.

To my question of 'What's made you the happiest?' the fathers' responses tended to be: the attainments of their sons and daughters against all the odds, and in direct contradiction to what they had been told at birth. Academic achievements featured highly, and the love of reading and language.

> 'Over dinner one night, my daughter was talking about "plates". We assumed she was talking about crockery, but she was referring to tectonic plates, as she had been learning all about earthquakes during geography!'

> 'My daughter is an excellent swimmer, and her coach gets her to show off her brilliant swimming technique

to other children in the swimming club. Who would have thought?'

'The pride at seeing my daughter in her gown when she graduated. Not to mention the speech she gave. I was in bits. We had a party with friends to celebrate, but I was too emotional to speak. She said to me, "It's all right, Dad. I'll do it."'

There was genuine surprise and delight that their children could be such great company when they grew older. 'My dream was always to share things with my children,' said one dad,

'and I can do this with her – the Down's makes no difference. I thought at first that she would be incredibly passive, and I would have to drag her along to cultural events. In fact, my experience is completely the opposite. We go to art galleries together, where she expresses her own unique opinions.'

Virtually every dad was proud of their child's personality and character: their sense of humour, their emotional intelligence and caring attitudes to people.

'My teenage son wants to shake hands with everyone, and loves children. He wants to pick them up, which sometimes frightens their mothers, and I have to explain, "It's OK, he's just being friendly."'

'My daughter isn't conditioned or socialised, and is simply connected to the core of humanity. She is so honest – everything comes straight from the heart, and so she lives in the "here and now". She is adventurous, creative and tells me, "I'm living the dream again. Today is very exciting . . . tomorrow will be even more exciting." She's fulfilled and genuinely happy in her own skin.'

'My daughter is full of humour, and has superb comic timing. She says the most normal things at the most bizarre times, and the most bizarre things at the most normal of times. She has made me feel intense pleasure and pain in equal measure.'

Not insignificantly, when I asked for some humorous stories, this brought forth the most material! Down's syndrome and comedy: two of my favourite subjects – and the combination is irresistible. Here are some of the best stories:

'My daughter often repeats film dialogue, and is a great mimic. We once got a frantic call from the school's speech and language therapist to say, "When your daughter comes home and tells you that I've been haranguing and accosting her, I really haven't! Honestly! Please believe me."

'When she got home, we asked her what happened. It transpired that when she had come out of the session, she picked up a telephone and said into it, "This woman's accosting me . . . this woman's accosting me!" and put the phone down. The therapist had heard the commotion and saw our girl walking down the corridor. She had actually been repeating dialogue from one of the *Home Alone* films, and the therapist naturally assumed she had been phoning home to make a complaint about her.'

'When my son was aged eight, we were in McDonald's. Sitting alone was a tattooed, shaven-headed bloke with two ferocious looking pit bulls under the table. My boy sat right opposite him, and took over the table, crowding the bloke out. I wasn't sure what was going to happen, and didn't fancy confronting him if it went off.

'The bloke looked up from his Big Mac, glanced at my lad, and said, 'All right, mate?', before returning to his grub. My boy melts hearts wherever he goes – he has an amazing effect on people.'

'My daughter is very vocal and chatty. She saw a some-what large lady and enquired, 'Why are you so fat?' My wife and I were horrified, and tried to shush her and move her away from the obese woman, but she had to have the last word, and exited triumphantly with a parting shot in earshot of, 'I bet that lady likes pizza.'

'We're big West Ham fans. I took my son to Everton a few years ago, and we had seats in the front row. Before kick-off, a woman who must have worked for 'Everton in the Community' saw him and said that they were inviting four fans from each side to take part in a half-time coaching session. We were close to the Everton fans, and there was lots of banter between us.

'At half-time, when my son went onto the pitch, he walked slowly past the Everton fans. My daughter was with me, and at the same time we both suddenly realised too late what was going to happen. Head down, my lad walked past gave the Everton fans and gave them the "wanker" sign! Of course, the West Ham fans loved it and cheered him. The Everton fans didn't know what to do. I think they were amused too, but in any case they couldn't really boo a boy with Down's syndrome.

'We were also at Millwall - the lower tier was kept empty for safety reasons, but as the players were coming out, my son needed the disabled toilet, which was pitch side by the corner flag in the Millwall section. We were accompanied by a steward, who then disappeared. When we came out of the toilet, my son sang, 'We're Forever Blowing Bubbles', and crossed his arms in the 'Hammers Salute' in front of all the Millwall fans. You can imagine how that went down! Unfortunately, the stewards wouldn't let us back to our seats and we had to sit on our own in the empty stand while getting plenty of abuse from the Millwall fans. Finally, a couple of coppers came to our rescue. My lad's absolutely fearless.'

'While at primary school, our daughter had attended an event with the children's writer, Michael Rosen. Some weeks later, at a local bookshop, she saw Raymond Briggs scribbling in some books. She approached him and told him that he shouldn't be writing in books.

"But I'm here to sign books – I'm an author," he said, defending himself.

A Major Adjustment

"No, you're not an author," she responded. "Michael Rosen is an author."'

(Raymond Briggs apparently stoically agreed.)

'Our daughter went to stay with some friends whose grandmother was suffering from dementia. She went into the room the elderly lady was occupying, danced with her and made the old girl laugh. When she came out of the room, she said, "I like her, but she's absolutely off her rocker!"'

'We'd been for a walk in a park. We were nearly back at the car when we came across an old man with a beard and a walking stick. My son ran up to him, grabbed him by the hand and greeted him like some long-lost friend. I obviously apologised to the old man, and asked my boy to let go of his hand, but the old man was overjoyed, and said it was the nicest thing that had happened to him for years.

Eventually we parted, and my son sat on a log and sighed happily. Then he gestured towards the old man and said, "Santa".

Who knows? He may have been right.

Another time we were at my mother's 80th birthday party – a BBQ held in the garden, although there were a few old people sitting inside. There was one rather frail old man called John, who was wheeled in by the womenfolk and put in a corner on his own. My boy liked him, so I checked that was OK with John and left them together for a while. Whilst I was in the garden I noticed my lad was being kept busy by the old folk collecting food and taking it back inside. However, when I nipped in to get a drink I discovered John, covered in about a dozen sausages, chicken legs and a lamb chop. He had no plate, so my son had just piled them onto his lap.'

'My daughter was invited to party at her godfather's smart buffet lunch. She has coeliac disease and, having been shown what she could and couldn't eat at the buffet table, she was then asked by the host to show another guest, who also had coeliac's, what *she* could eat from the buffet. She later found herself with her 'coeliac sister' and two other guests. They were a gay couple that she had met before but couldn't remember their names, but felt compelled to play the hostess and introduce them. She pointed at herself and said, "You know me . . . this is um . . . err . . . Gluten-free, and this is . . . um . . . um . . . Lesbian and Lesbian."'

One family were at a swimming pool whilst on holiday. Their five-year-old son fell off a bench in the changing room and hit the back of his head. They took him the local A&E, and discovered his skull had been fractured. He had always hit his head when he got frustrated – obviously now dangerous – and so from now on had to wear a bicycle helmet to protect himself.

The trouble was that the youngster wouldn't wear it unless his dad donned the same protective headgear. Every night on his return from work, therefore, his father would also have to wear a helmet, and so the two of them lounged around the house like exiles from the Tour de France.

Sadly, there is still much ignorance about Down's syndrome. One father told me about a friend of his with a child with DS who was in a queue at his local supermarket with his wife and son, and found a woman glancing nervously at their son. After further staring, the woman pointed at the young boy and asked, 'Is it catching?'

His mother fixed the woman with a hard look. 'Yes,' she replied, 'very. I expect you've probably got it by now.'

The fathers' hopes and fears for the future were pretty similar: first, a stoical acknowledgement that their sons and daughters will never be fully independent, and will always need some support to various degrees, not least in a continuing battling for funding. Then, because of the vulnerability of their offspring, worrying about their safety, and also wanting them to be in an inclusive community with a social network and lasting friendships. And then, hoping for happiness, fulfilment in work and play, long-term relationships and marriage – although these are the same for a parent of any child. There was a feeling of wanting their children to live with them for as long as possible, to provide a 'cocoon from rest of the world'. But there was a conundrum, for at the same time these fathers also wanted their offspring to be within their own community, where they could lead their own lives. One dad said, 'I just hope that she'll be smiling in the same way she does at 16.'

But, without exception, the overwhelming concern for the future was what would happen to their children when they and their partners were no longer around. And what part the siblings would play – a delicate balance of hoping and wanting their other children to do all they could, but not expecting them to feel responsible. It was hoped that the love between them was such that they would always want to be involved, and wouldn't feel burdened.

The bond between father and daughter is unique, and none more so than that between Anne de Gaulle, the youngest daughter of General Charles de Gaulle and his wife Yvonne, who was born 1928 with Down's syndrome. Her parents refused to place her in an institution, and Anne travelled everywhere with them. The usually undemonstrative future French president wanted to show her that he loved her as much as her two siblings, and would play and dance with and sing to Anne as much as he could, to the extent that their relationship was described as 'unconditional love between father and daughter.'

Anne died in 1948, aged 20, and the de Gaulles created an institution in her name, Fondation Anne de Gaulle. There are three establishments near Versailles that still provide care for adults with learning disabilities. 'Without Anne,' her father once said, 'I would never perhaps have done what I did. She gave me the heart and the inspiration.'

On 22 August 1962 the General was the target of an attempted assassination. Twelve men opened fire at his Citroën as it sped down the Avenue de la Libération in Paris, but their timing was off, and they started firing too late, with most of their bullets hitting the Citroën from behind, shattering the rear window. The car manufacturer later claimed the attempt was foiled by the car's futuristic, aerodynamic body design and superior mobility, which enabled the chauffeur to speed away to safety.

There is, however, another version of de Gaulle's escape which I prefer. According to the General, the potentially fatal bullet (it must have just been one of the 70) was stopped by the frame of the photograph of Anne he always carried with him – this time placed on the rear shelf of his car.

It's a wonderful story, and obviously apocryphal – but, should this book upset a particularly vengeful reader, I'm thinking of placing a framed photograph of Sarah in my left breast-pocket . . . just in case.

UNIQUE STEREOTYPES

In an excluded place and thy alone and not
worrying about being different everything is blissful
I can be alternative without the media change me I
can be old-school. And not think about my image
I can be in control I can punch my anger out I
can control the cursed words by the man. I can be
joyful my music is not popular. And I don`t care its
Punk Pop, Rock and old school pop I don`t need
to worry about not being model like beauty is skin
deep and that's why I stay in my room.

Jess Hardie, 'In My Bedroom'

In 2003, Sarah became involved in an innovative and imaginative project that involved friends of hers who just happened to have Down's syndrome, and their parents, who just happened to be photographers. Shifting Perspectives was a group of seven photographers – Richard and Fiona Bailey, Fiona Yaron-Field, Aviv Yaron, Maria de Fatima Campos, Kayte Brimacombe and Richard Davis – who realised that photographs of people with Down's tended to depict them as very much institutionalised – white tube socks and pudding-basin haircuts – and weren't an accurate depiction of people with the condition. So they set out to challenge attitudes and prejudices by representing both adults and children in a different way.

The first exhibition was held in a local café for Down's Syndrome Awareness Week, and one of the visitors was Susan Andrews, a senior lecturer from London Metropolitan University, who asked the group if they would like to participate in 'Photomonth', which was held in the East End every year. An exhibition was subsequently held at the university, curated by Susan, and featured on BBC Radio 4's *Front Row*. 'We live in an era where "image is everything,"' Susan wrote,

> and as such the power attributed to the photograph is immense and in many ways vitally important. It not only determines our perception of the appearance of the individual but also implies their personality and situation. The photographers investigate their worlds as questioning artists, aware of the representation and photographic genre, each with a very personal vision.

One of the earliest projects conceived by Richard and Fiona Bailey was '365', photographing 365 children, one for every day of the year, dressing the subjects identically in black T-shirts, and arranging the 10 x 8 prints together in a 6 x 3-metre rectangle that covered a wall. As Susan Andrews explains, 'the juxtaposition of identically displayed photographs reveals not uniformity, but character and individuality.'

In 2005, the collective exhibited for the first time at the Oxo Tower's gallery on London's South Bank, and the exhibition, supported by GlaxoSmithKline, was a resounding success. The response was unprecedented in numerous ways: people with

Unique Stereotypes

Down's syndrome were delighted to see images that at last portrayed them accurately; to their parents it gave a feeling of community, and a sense of all that a new-born baby with Down's could have achieved long ago; and those without a link to disability were drawn simply to the vibrant images, and found their awareness about the condition increased.

Each year the exhibition had a new theme, including employment, culture, beliefs and desires, marriage and relationships, and subsequently the group expanded to 11 photographers. Among the portraits taken by Richard Bailey was one of the ubiquitous Sarah Gordy called 'After Vermeer', in which he reconstructed Vermeer's encounters with his sitters. 'Sarah's grace, charm and character were perfect to emulate Vermeer's elegant studies,' said Bailey – 'but with a modern twist.'

In 2011 Fiona Yaron-Field exhibited 'Safe Haven', a series of photos of pregnant women who knew their babies would be born with Down's syndrome and had, unusually, decided to carry the baby to full term (92 per cent of women will abort a foetus with Down's syndrome). 'Maybe I do have some need to expose the myths and stereotypes about Down's syndrome that are deeply engraved in society's consciousness,' Fiona writes. 'These stereotypes, which can be either positive or negative, are one-dimensional, and dismiss the complexity and depth that people experience both with themselves and in relation to others. They deny the person any "real identity".'

Shifting Perspectives has since been seen in over 50 venues in 12 different countries, and there are currently plans to exhibit at the 2020 Tokyo Olympic and Paralympic Games. The project also featured some guest photographers with DS, and the response was so positive that in 2010 the Down's Syndrome Association decided to launch a national competition to highlight unrecognised talent, and provide a means for photographers with Down's to share their images. My Perspective is now an annual exhibition.

Sarah was also involved in an 'edgy' integrated arts and photography project. Joel accompanied Sarah to her shoot at the BOY/GIRL studio in Lewisham. There they found, he recalls, an

> incredibly vibrant atmosphere, and the photographers, Liz and Jason, and their stylist addressed Sarah's every need – obviously her outfit, hair, and make-up, but also her music requests on Spotify! I was acting as chaperone, but I felt like Sarah's special guest at this *Vogue*-like photoshoot. It was a thoroughly enjoyable experience for both of us, and one of the very favourite times I have spent with Sarah. They were all so lovely, and embodied the generation that has accepted people with Down's syndrome in recent times.

The result of the shoot was an extraordinarily striking black and white photograph of Sarah, adorned in a Gothic cloak and feathers and sporting an elaborate Mohican hair style. She had always refused to wear make-up, but so completely trusted the team working around her that she agreed to some cosmetic adornment. Her reaction when she saw her portrait was 'Wow! I love it.' We all did – it was such a cutting-edge, dramatic image, and so removed from the idiom in which adults with Down's syndrome were usually depicted.

'Children and adults with Down's syndrome need to be accepted in all areas of everyday life,' I wrote in 1999 in *A Minor Adjustment*, and they must be seen to be part of society – not outside it. Advertising plays an important part in creating trends by portraying normal, family life, and it is only recently that, apart from the Benetton advertisement the odd charitable organisation and a Mothercare catalogue from nearly ten years ago, I have never seen a child or person with Down's syndrome encouraging the sale of a particular product on television or in a magazine. Is this because the image is too negative? Would the appearance of a child with learning disabilities really turn people off from buying clothes, breakfast cereals or toys?

Things are slowly changing. Caroline White is a powerful advocate for inclusion, who with her son Seb is patron of an organisation called the Musicman Project, a theatre group for adults with learning disabilities, and in 2012 her son Seb was the first model with Down's to star in a major UK television advertisement, for M&S. 'My drive for him to model was based on many things,' explains Caroline:

> inclusion and representation, mainly. I remember vividly, when he was a baby, seeing a Waitrose television advertisement that featured a giant picnic blanket and hundreds of families. I knew there wouldn't be one that represented my family. At a time of feeling 'different' and isolated, it made me feel worse. I had emailed and emailed many retailers and modelling agents and either been fobbed off or ignored, so I took to Facebook and posted my plea. M&S listened and called him in for a shoot. He did so well that they then invited him to be in the TV ad.

A Major Adjustment

Caroline has also written a book, *The Label*, a fable based on her real experience, which in the autumn of 2017 was adapted into a musical and performed as part of a larger show at the London Palladium.

In the same year, several children with Down's were selected to appear in advertising campaigns. In Ireland Abby Dillon has become the face of Glenisk's Organic baby yoghurts. Lilly Bedall, aged two, won a modelling contract with the fashion retailer Matalan, resulting in her picture being exhibited in every one of the chain's 217 UK stores. Even more recently, Joseph Hale, an 11-year-old boy with Down's syndrome from Grimsby, landed his first official modelling job as part of River Island's latest children's advertising campaign. 'Advertising can put across in a very positive way, that even if a person has a special need and/or a disability, they still have emotions, thoughts, feelings, and dreams the same as anyone else,' his parents Karen and Andrew were quoted as saying.

> The impact of more brands including mixed abilities in advertising could be huge – not just for our son, but for anyone with a special need and/or a disability . . . individuals would see that his disability doesn't define him, and that there are still many more amazing layers of him to discover.

In October 2017 a teenager with Down's made her catwalk debut at Belfast Fashion Week. Kate Grant, from County Tyrone, was 'discovered' when her mother Deirdre posted an image of her on Facebook, describing her daughter's desire to work in the fashion industry, and adding that she wanted to challenge perceptions of beauty and shine a light on discrimination faced by those with a disability: 'She has the same aspirations as any other girl who wants to be a model. . . Please support her. Just maybe her dreams will come true.' Within a week the Facebook post had gone viral, and resulted in the 19-year-old model receiving a standing ovation when she posed confidently at the event in St Anne's Cathedral.

Seeing more and more children and adults with Down's syndrome being represented in all parts of our society must help in tackling, and eventually eliminating, the negative, pre-conceived ideas the majority of people still have about the condition. As Johann Wolfgang von Goethe said, 'The way you see people is the way you treat them, and the way you treat them is what they become.'

11

A COLLEGE KID

Tell me and I forget. Teach me and I remember.
Involve me and I learn.

Benjamin Franklin

Although Sarah had managed the equivalent of four GSCE passes, A-levels were not for her. For the prospect of future employment, she needed to pursue a more practical path, and so continued her post- 16 education initially in 'life skills', and then on a City & Guilds course in food studies, hospitality and catering at the local sixth-form college. Her statement of special educational needs remained in effect, so she continued to receive extra support when she transferred in September 2008.

Haringey Sixth-Form College was a brand new centre in Tottenham, only recently opened (again our timing was perfect): a state-of-the-art building, all chrome and glass and buzzing with hundreds of noisy, vibrant and exuberant urban teenagers. Sarah had been happy in her two local schools, where she knew lots of people and had been quite protected, but this was a different challenge altogether. While we were daunted at Sarah being in a totally new environment, Sarah, with her accustomed courage, rose to the challenge and, although a little nervous, settled in very quickly. There was also a bonus in that Liz, one of the teaching staff from her secondary school, who had a nephew with Down's, now worked at the college and was very helpful in the transition.

Allie and I had to adjust to Sarah's new-found freedom and growing independence. After some 'travel training', Sarah started taking the local W3 bus route, and travelled to school on her own. In the early days we quietly panicked, worrying that she might travel in the wrong direction, not alight at the right stop, become completely lost and disorientated, and then, of course, don't think the possibility of her being kidnapped hadn't crossed our minds.

In fact, we needn't have concerned ourselves, as her commuting mainly went smoothly, although there was one occasion when she didn't hear the bus driver's instruction of 'Everybody off!' at one of the stops, and ended up as the sole passenger at the terminus. Up on the top deck she hadn't realised what was happening, and duly received a sound telling-off from the driver. She might well have spent the night in the bus station if he hadn't checked that his transport was empty. But Sarah recovered her confidence, and became a big fan of her local bus route. In fact, we were once on a holiday in Croatia, enjoying a boat trip between the islands, basking in the sunshine and stunning scenery, when Allie asked Sarah if she was enjoying herself. With total sincerity, Sarah replied, 'I prefer being on the W3.'

Apart from specific classes, there were lots of other activities that Sarah enjoyed and which helped her integrate into college life. A few months into her first term, Sarah wrote about her new life.

My first day at Haringey sixth form centre I was a bit nervous but now am not because I made friends. we are having lots of fun like lea valley rowing club and football or cooking. I am so excited this year! Today we went to see Judo at the showcase at wood green that was awesome. I like it here sometimes we do sports altogether its great and of course we do cycling I learnt how to cycle as well. and I learnt how to row. now I am great at it so that's my life ahead of me

In her second year, Sarah took a City & Guilds Entry-Level Certificate in Food Studies, studying health, safety and hygiene, learning about the importance of a balanced diets, and doing food prep and cooking. She was also taught about 'front of house' and food service. 'Without fail Sarah is the first student to arrive for her classes,' read her end-of-year report,

whether they be in the classroom, kitchen or restaurant. She will always work hard, is enthusiastic in all that she does and is a pleasure to have around and to teach. She does, however, sometimes lack confidence and is afraid to make mistakes in case she looks 'stupid' in front of her class. But she will always encourage others to do their best.

It was true that Sarah's self-belief, which had hitherto been completely solid, was at times tested. She had always hated letting people down and, now she was working in a team, this responsibility weighed heavily on her. 'Sarah can be very sensitive at times,' commented her inspirational mentor at the college, Dawn Taylor,

and this can have a negative impact on her self-esteem and how she works in class. She is a very capable

student who would benefit from trusting herself more
. . . when Sarah makes a mistake, especially in the
kitchen, it almost seems that her world has come to
an end. However, she has made some very successful
mistakes in cooking and her work has turned out
well!

The class provided and served food in the college restaurant,
and Sarah began to discover her true vocation, to the extent that
Dawn wrote, 'Sarah has dealt remarkably well with front-of-
house pressures. Customers have commented on the quality of
customer service that she has provided, and she takes a great deal
of pride in her work.'

During her second year, Sarah stood as class representative
and, with some help, wrote an election statement.

First, I'd like to say that I'm really enjoying being a
member of the colleagues' class. I want to be your
class representative because I am very positive about
this class. It will make my dream come true if the
colleagues vote for me because I never had this in my
life. I will talk to the other students and the teachers,
of course and will represent your views at all times. I
will always ask for your ideas and opinions. And I am
very firm and strong. It would be awesome to be your
rep – so please vote for me It will make me very happy.

I'm delighted to say Sarah was duly elected as class representative,
without having to kiss any babies or the involvement of President
Putin. She undertook her responsibilities dutifully and with a glad
heart. Her first election promise was to obtain a door for the

classroom. This surprised us – not just her practical and sensible policy, but that there wasn't already a door in situ.

The year of 2010 also saw Sarah vote for the first time, in the May General Election of that year. I had written about voting in *A Minor Adjustment*, long before Sarah would be eligible to vote.

> When Sarah reaches the age of 18, I would hope that she has the same opportunity to exert her democratic right as everybody else and, in this way, make a contribution to the political system that makes laws about what she can and cannot do. I feel sure that if Sarah continues to absorb as much knowledge as she has been, and the issues are explained to her in a straightforward and clear manner, she would be quite able to decide whom to vote for.

We encouraged Sarah to participate in an online election questionnaire that advised the participant which political party was most suited to their political opinions. We simplified some of the more complex questions for her, and at the end of the survey Sarah's answers fitted the bill of a Labour Party voter. And to confirm her political philosophy, Sarah later declared, 'I'm going to vote Labour in any case because I met Sarah Brown and I like her.'

Sarah was very excited on 6 May, and we all went off to the polling station together. On the way Allie and I were suddenly concerned that Sarah, alone in the booth, would call out, 'Mum! Dad! Who did you say I should vote for?' Officials would be called, the Labour candidate would be suspended, there'd be a recount in the constituency, and the whole election would be called null and void because of Sarah. Fortunately, she discharged her democratic right with the minimum of fuss and a cross correctly placed on the ballot paper. The election result stood, though, which was a bit of a shame.

I've always enjoyed elections. I remember once, when 'telling' for the Labour Party, the policewoman on duty, who bore an uncanny resemblance to Joyce Grenfell, both in looks and manner, suggesting we try and convince her to vote for our selected parties. The blue-rinsed Tory lady, with whom I had been getting on famously, explained amicably to our own Sgt Ruby Gates that one of her responsibilities while on duty at the polling station was to stop us from doing exactly that. 'Oh,' she said. 'What a twit I am.'

In the spring of 2010, slap-bang in the middle of Sarah's three years at the Sixth-Form College, the comedian Frankie Boyle caused quite a stir in the Down's syndrome community – not to mention the Merriman household.

Kieron Smith and his wife Sharon went to the Hexagon Theatre in Reading for the opening night of the Scottish comic's tour. Counting themselves fans of his, the couple were prepared for some cutting, scathing humour, and had got seats in the front row. Then Boyle launched into a routine which targeted people with Down's syndrome, joked about early death, bad haircuts and clothes, the age and dowdiness of their parents, and even attempted to mimic in an incomprehensible, puerile voice how a 'Mongoloid' speaks. Sharon, the mother of Tanzie, their daughter with Down's, then five years old, became increasingly uncomfortable.

Kieron asked her if she was OK. Boyle noticed, and asked why they were talking during his show. Sharon told him that she had a daughter with Down's, and was naturally upset.

'This could be the most excruciating moment of my career,' responded the comic, but then added, 'But it's all true, isn't it?'

To which the Smiths replied, no, it wasn't.

Frankie Boyle never apologised, and the following morning, in response to questions from her friends, Sharon posted a blog, describing what happened and how she felt. There followed an interview in the *Guardian* and coverage in most national newspapers, and media interest on television and radio news.

'To the audience I was just "some woman who got offended,"' Sharon wrote on her blog.

> I wish that I had managed to explain to them all why I was upset, to tell them how wrong the stereotypes about Down syndrome are. I wanted to show them how proud I am of my daughter, how beautiful and intelligent she is, to tell them how well she is doing at mainstream school . . . but instead all I did was to make people think I was someone who couldn't appreciate live stand-up comedy, which isn't the case at all.

Frankie Boyle was messing with the wrong family. Aside from Sharon's response, Kieron has written an authoritative book, *The Politics of Down Syndrome,* in which he examines all aspects of the condition, and provides a historical and philosophical approach to the subject. 'Down syndrome seems to have transformed into a metaphor,' he writes in it,

> a metaphor primarily for stupidity, whereby words such as 'Mong', 'a Down's', 'Retard', are able to become an easy insult, a shared 'other' which represents idiocy and contempt. These terms represent a diminution of people with DS to something akin to sub-humanity.

A College Kid

Kieron sent Frankie Boyle a copy of his book but, unsurprisingly, didn't receive a response.

The DSA responded to the incident by repeating a campaign it had used 25 years earlier: a very successful nationwide poster campaign, with the strapline,

YOU SAY MONGOL.

WE SAY DOWN'S SYNDROME.

HIS MATES CALL HIM DAVID.

As someone who had a foot in both the comedy and the disability camps, I was asked to appear on Sky News. In a brief interview, I said that I felt very little should be considered 'off-limits' for comedy, and performing dangerous material wasn't a new thing. Lenny Bruce had, after all, been banned by the Home Secretary from entering the UK back in the 1960s – but the big difference was that Bruce was funny and tackled hypocrisy and cant, whereas Boyle's so-called routine was nothing more than an abusive rant and based on 1950s stereotypes. And of course, the biggest misdemeanour a comedian can commit while being abusive is being unfunny . . . and this was very unfunny.

We were all pretty upset, but Sarah was really incensed, and, without prompting from us, announced that she wanted to write to the Glaswegian comic.

Dear FRANKIE BOYLE

Look here – tell me why do you hate down syndrome people we haven't done anything wrong I know its your work being a stand up comedian but its not that funny at all I have down syndrome so what? That is part of me and I am not going on about it so please tell me why you found this hilarious. I am not pleased at all. you are in the wrong here. We are who we are. understand that or should we say you're not a very charming man.

PS I am not complaining about it. I am very proud of myself. That's just me!

SARAH MERRIMAN

We posted the letter to the comedian's agent, but of course, never heard back. The following year Ofcom censured Boyle for his jokes about the TV celebrity Katie Price's disabled son. 'I once saw Frankie Boyle sitting by the window in a café,' one of the dads I interviewed told me. 'I knocked on the glass and, when Boyle looked up, I gave him two fingers – I don't suppose he had a clue why I did it, but it made me happy.'

Meanwhile, back in Tottenham, Sarah's college mentor, Dawn Taylor, was reporting that

Sarah works hard in the kitchen, but it is front of house that is her strength, she needs something that will build on this. Yes, Sarah has special needs, but she is living in a world that is not special needs and she is functioning and learning to cope quite well. Sarah is capable of holding down a job, and with the right support she will do that.

A College Kid

To this end, Sarah obtained some work experience. She spent a week at her old primary school, helping the teaching and support staff with young children in the classroom; a week at the DSA, assisting with administration tasks; and two weeks at a nursery, helping staff in feeding, supervising, and playing with the children. But the most successful placement was another fortnight, this time at a day centre for older people, where she helped prepare and serve meals. Amazingly, at the end of the fortnight she was offered a permanent, full-time paid job as a kitchen assistant. But she was desperate to go to college, and so we had to decline the offer. But we were thrilled to know that she had done so well, and employment in the future wasn't just a pipe dream.

Sarah was due to complete her time at sixth-form college in June 2011, and her biggest challenge now lay ahead. It was time for us to think about life for her beyond Haringey, and plans were now required for her next institute of learning. All being well, she would complete her City & Guilds course at Entry 3 level, and we wanted her to continue in catering and hospitality, where she could progress to the next level. There were a number of objectives to be taken into consideration in her next placement: developing Sarah's communication skills and friendships, building teamwork, and providing a safe and secure learning environment while enhancing her social skills.

But most important of all was that she needed the chance for of independent living – with support – and also meaningful employment. We were absolutely adamant that, just as Daniel had gone away to university, so Sarah should have the same opportunity to spread her wings away from home. How best to achieve this?

We were visited by Costas, a social worker from the social services transition team, and Sarah's 'Comprehensive Assessment' of her needs was initiated with regard to funding the next placement. Although now officially 'clients', we made it clear to Costas from the start that we had both been social workers (Allie still was) and, although empathising with his workload, we were well versed in the profession, which we felt would keep him on his mettle. We needn't have worried: he was very efficient and helpful, and interviewed Sarah in a very sympathetic manner. There were a few humorous moments, particularly when Costas showed Sarah a picture of an iron, and asked her what she might use it for.

'Don't know,' was her response. 'Never seen one.' I think that said much more about our levels of domesticity than Sarah's actual needs.

I must admit that the report's conclusions made somewhat depressing reading, and brought home to us how much Sarah would need in years to come.

> Requires support with reading and writing, with finances, including money management. No concept of budgeting, values or correct change. Needs help with independent travel, reminding and prompting about hygiene matters, and to develop life skills such as cooking, cleaning, washing up, laundry, and insight to reduce her vulnerability. Does not comprehend the severity or implications – lacks the sophistication of an 18-year-old. Very motivated and organised, she gets fretful about transitions but manages these well. She is not always understood, as she often speaks too fast, and tends to dominate conversation when in groups.
>
> She has no understanding of abstract concepts, and has limited comprehension, requiring people to speak slowly and deliberately, using concrete terms

and explanations. She also requires visual prompts and pictorial reinforcement (photos and symbols) – necessitated ongoing speech and language input. Difficulty with fine motor skills. Limited memory – especially short-term – and concentration is poor: frequent repetition is required. Copes better with organised activities.

Following the completion of her assessment, the local authority looked into several local colleges that Sarah could attend, which, in contrast to a residential setting, would obviously save it money. We understood the thinking: Haringey was strapped for cash. If one of these colleges was suitable for her, then we would consider the options, but we still felt very strongly that Sarah should be given a similar opportunity to her brother, who was at Sheffield University and living independently.

She also needed to be able to flee the nest, and it was even more imperative that she was working towards a life independent from us. With Dawn Taylor's guidance, we soon realised that none of the suggested local colleges would further Sarah's future independence or skills. One of these local colleges would not provide enough support, while at another she would be repeating most of the things she had already learned, and at a third, it was felt, she would be delegated all the menial tasks. None of them could offer as a holistic experience the training as well as development of independent living skills that Sarah needed.

But by now we had heard of Foxes Academy, a training hotel for learning-disabled young people in Somerset. It seemed perfect for Sarah and, although a little daunted about being so far from the family home, she was very keen to attend. We decided to set the bureaucratic wheels in motion.

A Major Adjustment

We were in contact with Connexions, formerly the Careers Service, a government organisation which offered information, advice, guidance and support up to the age of 25 for young people with learning difficulties and/or disabilities. (The coalition government's public spending cuts hit Connexions' services badly, and in many areas the service vanished altogether). We stressed Sarah's requirements to Jim, our Connexions worker, who, despite being an Arsenal fan, temporarily agreed to put aside our north London rivalry and proved crucially helpful in our quest to find the best possible provision for Sarah.

The agreement for funding seemed to take a very long time without any progress. Just at the point where we were becoming desperate – a mere few months before Sarah's place at Foxes had to be taken up – we were advised that funding had been agreed. What we hadn't realised was that, behind the scenes, Jim and Costas had been battling tirelessly on our behalf for a residential placement for Sarah, and had gone to the appropriate social services panel to put our case *nine times*.

When Sarah left the sixth-form college, she gave a speech to her class.

> I will be very sad to leave here. I have really enjoyed it. I loved this college, it's cool. So, I want to say a big thank you to these people: Kate and Epe: teachers in my first year. Thank you for supporting me and making this fun for me. You're so kind and I will miss both of you so much. Dawn and Connie: where do I begin? You've been brilliant to me for 2 years. You are both very special to me and I'm going to think about you all the time. And I will really miss you very much. Angela and Verity Thank you so much for helping

with my work and I will miss you loads. Martin, I
want to say thank you for being my special friend.
I will miss you so much and I loved your lessons on
Friday afternoons. And of course, all my friends.
Thank you everyone for your friendship and love.
I hope you will let me come and visit one day.

'Sarah has taught me so much about my job,' wrote Dawn
Taylor, 'so it really is a two-way thing. I truly believe that she has
given me far more than I have given her.'

Allie and I wrote to Haringey's Director of Children's Services
to say how much Sarah had benefited throughout her life from
the department's involvement, and through her attendance in
mainstream education, where she had been admirably supported
and made to feel so welcome by teachers and teaching assistants.
'In recent years,' we ended up, 'Haringey has received much
negative publicity, both nationally and locally, and so we wished to
address the balance by describing our own positive experiences.'

We sent copies to several local and a couple of national newspapers. None of them published our letter. I suppose good news
is no news.

12

MIND YOUR BACKS,
SHARP KNIFE COMING THROUGH

*Did you ever have the feeling that you wanted to
go, and then you had the feeling that you wanted
to stay?*

Jimmy Durante,
The Man Who Came to Dinner

I suppose, having penned the 'autobiography' of Basil Brush a few
years previously, it was somehow inevitable that I would find my
daughter ensconced at a place called Foxes Academy.

The Academy was founded in 1996 by Sue Jenkins and
Maureen Tyler-Moore, who were both working in a residential
care home and had become dispirited by the lack of resources and
opportunities for young people with learning disabilities. It only
needed the right level of training and support, they felt, for their
charges to reveal hitherto-untapped skills and talents which could
lead to them gaining meaningful employment. So they decided to
set up their own establishment.

After a search for the right premises the two women found
Westholme Hotel, on the seafront in the north Somerset resort
of Minehead. It dated back to 1886, and was originally built to
entertain the aristocracy and visiting Indian maharajas who came

to play polo at Dunster Castle. They named it Foxes Academy. To us its principal attraction was that it was both college and training hotel: its students, or 'learners', are employed in the working environment of a real hotel which is open to the public. In 2010 Sarah and I visited to see what we thought of the place.

We stayed in the hotel overnight to get a feel of the town, and as Sarah and I breakfasted there the next morning I watched the staff carefully to see how they related to the learners. I was immediately impressed by how they offered just the right assistance and support without patronising the learners in the slightest. The biggest impact, however, was made by our waitress. The young woman with Down's who served us was confident, efficient and friendly. When I tried to engage her in conversation Sarah was a little embarrassed, telling me the waitress had work to do and I shouldn't distract her. I wondered then if Sarah might one day be capable of similar employment, and whether she would ever be as professional as this Foxes student.

I immediately knew this was the place for Sarah, and rang Allie to tell her. The college seemed to offer everything Sarah needed – not only did it offer the training in catering, hospitality and general life skills Sarah needed, but the small seaside town of Minehead also offered a perfect environment for a city girl in exile. A sort of arcadian sanctum.

Although geographically somewhat isolated – the nearest mainline railway station, Taunton, is an hour's bus ride away – the advantage was that Minehead was far away enough for us not to be able to 'pop in' if we were anxious about Sarah. Though described as 'a dormitory for the elderly', the town was geared up for each year's influx of learners, and enjoyed a symbiotic relationship with the college: Foxes used Minehead's facilities and held events in various premises and, whereas some communities might be mistakenly nervous about hosting too many adults with learning disabilities, this town's people positively welcomed having learners and their families in their midst. Some of the shops had 'Safe Haven' stickers in their windows, so that Foxes students who became lost, disorientated or anxious could go in and explain their predicament. Foxes would then be contacted, and the learner could be 'rescued'.

Minehead's economy is dominated by the Butlin's holiday camp at the other end of town, which also had a good relationship with Foxes (other than during its 'Adult Weekends', when marauding, scantily-clad revellers sporting hideous fake appendages and boobs were kept at bay from the learners).

Some months later, Allie took Sarah down to Foxes, again staying overnight in the hotel, for her to be interviewed by several members of staff from various disciplines to assess her suitability. She very much enjoyed the experience, and was keen to be accepted. Allie, meanwhile, was bowled over by the professionalism and enthusiasm of the staff, and met some of the trainees. She remembers looking out of the window at the sea, across the hotel's sunny front lawn, where third-year learners were industriously preparing their end-of-term barbecue, and knowing then that Sarah would fit in perfectly.

When Sarah was younger there was something it always hurt me to think about: I would never be able to visit her at college, take her and some of her friends out to lunch, and hear all about their academic achievements – or at least which gig they had gone to and how drunk they had got the night before. She wouldn't share the experiences her brothers were likely to have. But now that was about to change. (In fact, Sarah hasn't actually ever touched a drop of alcohol. It's not that she's 'taken the pledge' or is some kind of killjoy: far from it. She just doesn't like the idea of even the tiniest snifter. We have on occasion thought of spiking her J2O, just to see if she could take her normal exuberance and merry-making to a new level, but have so far resisted the temptation.)

Sarah started at Foxes in September 2011. As the date to leave home approached she became more anxious, but kept telling us that 'I must be strong.' When the time came to travel down to Somerset we took the boys along – they both wanted to see where Sarah was going, and spend as much time with her as possible up to the moment when she officially left home.

The night before we were due to leave her we stayed in a pub in nearby Washford, coincidentally the same village where my dad had been stationed with the RAF during the war. As we approached Minehead the next morning Sarah began blubbing, which set us all off, although we also 'wanted to be strong' as we tried to comfort her. She knew it was the right thing, and that she was ready to move away from home, but now the reality was hitting her.

But it wasn't long before we were unpacking in her lovely attic room in Foxes Den, a house in the high street she was to share with six other learners, and then an extremely hunky young man walked past Sarah's open door – he was occupying the room next door. Allie and I looked at one another, both delighted and terrified. . .

We left quickly before we were all reduced to quivering wrecks and, instead of exploring the rolling Somerset countryside as we had planned to do, decided to drive home straight away. The thought of being so near to an unhappy Sarah was painful enough, but not being able to comfort her was unbearable.

The first phone call wasn't long in coming. That evening, Sarah rang us. She was already homesick, miserable, she missed us and wanted to come home. Allie spoke to a member of staff who, although sympathetic, dissuaded us from even thinking about coming to see Sarah. We resisted the temptation of becoming too involved so early on, and didn't want to undermine the staff. Previous visits to Foxes had given us the confidence that they knew exactly what they were doing.

After about two weeks, Sarah rang again. Her gloom had turned into annoyance, because until the staff got to know her, she wasn't being allowed the freedom she had at home. 'I'm pissed off. And so is my friend Freddie. We are adults. And they won't allow us outside on our own. I'm going to talk to the staff!'

Sarah was kicking against the rules. We wondered initially whether we might have placed Sarah in an environment where her independence would be restricted. However, speaking with a staff member, reassured us of the context for such rules: before new students could be granted further freedoms, a 'risk assessment' had to take place. Sarah's exasperation signalled a turning-point in her confidence about being away from us. Over the next few weeks she became much happier in her new, stimulating environment, and began not only to grapple with a new-found independence, but also to thoroughly enjoy herself.

Sarah came home for the Christmas holidays, and it was lovely to have her back. Daniel was in his second year at Sheffield, and it seemed that Sarah was doing just the same as him – studying away at college. Of course, the circumstances were different and, although a degree in politics and history would certainly do him no harm, it wouldn't, unlike Sarah's course, set him up with a vocation or a job. Sarah was already learning more about food service, catering skills and the philosophy of healthy eating. Although it must be said that her dire warnings of the dangers of cross-contamination and cry of 'Mind your backs, sharp knife coming through!' – echoing with great seriousness Foxes' chef Helen – got short shrift from her two brothers, indeed provoked only mirth, much to Sarah's indignation.

At the end of the first year, Sarah received a report from Nina, her house manager and Residential Life co-ordinator.

> Sarah is a lovely, polite and able young lady. She has made incredible progress this year and matured into an independent young woman. She has developed good friendships with her peers, and is very considerate towards others. She can be emotional when she encounters difficult situations – needs reassurance and positive advice to help her deal with the issues bothering her. She is very good at taking advice and will accept help from staff – she likes having a joke with staff and peers.

Sarah wrote an article by herself, 'My Life at Foxes', for *Down2Earth* magazine, describing her first year and activities.

> When I started here in foxes I felt nervous about the new changes. Afterwards I said to myself I love it here in foxes so when I felt really happy because I started doing housekeeping I cleaned the toilets and bed-rooms. Also I did food preparation I discovered that I really enjoyed it. Also serving all the guests and working as a team. also I do a lot of clubs. I love doing the Zumba that is really fun. I played football in the west community college I really enjoyed it. Trampolining I do this every Wednesdays. Drama last term we all made up Oliver twist for our xmas panto

I was a Fagin boy that was really fun and we did that in Butlins everyone was watching it. Healthy eating. To stay healthy. Skills for life we do all sorts of things like using the computer and how to stay safe. Whenever I am down or upset I go and get the staff to help me with it. My whole life in foxes is been a new experience for me.

I LOVE IT

Sarah couldn't have been happier, and entered her second year with gusto. She was developing her skills in catering and hospitality by working in the kitchen and housekeeping sections of the hotel, and gained hugely from the discipline of a working environment. Equally important was Sarah's progress in independent living. She was learning how to budget; her personal hygiene was much improved; her domestic abilities were developing out of all recognition – whenever Allie visited, she found Sarah's room to be beautifully clean and tidy. (Sarah used to speak proudly of her 'deep cleaning' method – something to which our family have always been strangers.) She did her own laundry and ironing, suggested ideas for menus, and was generally becoming more organised in her day-to-day living.

Sharing a house (now with eight other young adults) in a supported environment helped her immeasurably in being able to share responsibilities in cooking and domestic duties, and negotiate the challenges of living with others as peers. Sarah found the earlier transitions back and forth from home to Foxes quite difficult, but began to integrate both areas of her life, focusing on the positive aspects of each. The staff at Foxes were excellent. They consistently encouraged the learners to be independent, but were always supportive when they met with any difficulties or problems.

Mind Your Backs, Sharp Knife Coming Through

During Sarah's third year the staff felt that, in readiness for more independent living, she should move into a bedsit in one of their houses, where she could be more self-contained, and even prepare her own food. A room was found for her at the top of Foxes Court.

The move was well-intentioned, but Sarah, wanting always to be at the hub of things, felt isolated, and didn't cook for herself properly, as she still needed supervision to prepare even the simplest meal. It also didn't help that the fridge was literally at the bottom of her bed, which was just too tempting for late-night unhealthy snacks and drinks. She struggled to cope, and soon moved into a downstairs bedroom in the house. It was useful to have had the opportunity for her to experience bedsit living, but too much of a challenge for her at that time.

Sarah did continue to progress in many other aspects, however, gaining in emotional maturity and increasing in confidence with work skills and personal organisation – taking medication, for example. However, her competence with money remained very limited: she was still unable to understand the value of money, or even recognise different coins.

She began work experience in the Combe training restaurant at West Somerset Community College and received very positive feedback.

> Sarah has a very professional attitude to her work and endeavours to complete all tasks to the best of her ability. She is enthusiastic and eager, and works hard within the team to spur on those around her. . . Sarah's strengths definitely lie with her customer-care skills, recording of orders and communicating with guests.

A Major Adjustment

As the time for Sarah to leave Foxes drew nearer, she became very sad at the thought of moving on, and understandably anxious. It was hard for her to imagine anywhere else that could offer her the same level of security, stimulation and happiness. And she was going to miss her fellow learners: one of her closest friends at Foxes was an excellent swimmer and cyclist, who was selected for the British Special Olympic cycling team to go to Los Angeles in 2015. Another pal, Anna, is a young woman Sarah still sees regularly, and whose parents are now our friends. Freddie was a real character, a charming young man who on one occasion was meant to be serving us breakfast, but instead entertained us with a sort of 20-minute stand-up routine. Another time, Sarah pointed out a young woman clad in dungarees sporting a short, spiky hairstyle. 'That's Jane', said Sarah, before adding nonchalantly, 'She's lesbian and likes people to know.' And then there was Hetty, one of Sarah's housemates, who, when Sarah introduced me, remarked, 'Oh, you're meant to be the famous writer. . . Well, I've never heard of you!'

I was tempted to respond with, 'Well, I've never heard of you,' but of course I had heard a lot about Hetty, and particularly her trips with Sarah to the Hairy Dog pub, a favourite haunt of the Foxes learners.

Just before Midsummer's Day 2014, Sarah attended a demonstration outside the Houses of Parliament. It wasn't her first, and I'm certain it won't be her last, but for her and her friends it couldn't have been more important. This protest was the dignified launch of A Right, Not a Fight – a campaign to highlight the need for educational equality for disabled people, which was supported by specialist colleges from all over the country. Sarah had travelled by coach from Somerset in the company of fellow students and staff from Foxes. I also went along, and it was impossible not to be moved by the dignity, confidence and earnestness of the students outside Westminster as they talked proudly of their achievements and their hopes for the future.

Around this time, specialist colleges like Foxes, along with their umbrella organisation Natspec and parents' groups and charities, had been providing input on the then new Children and Families Act, to ensure that every young person could get the education they deserved. One of the act's key principles is, quite simply, to listen to the views and wishes of the young people themselves and their parents. It also enshrines in law the principle that students with a physical or learning disability should have the same choices most young people take for granted – like choosing a further education college that best meets their needs.

Young people with physical or learning disabilities face particular challenges and difficulties with education and employment. While it may be possible for them to work and live independently, they sometimes take longer to learn new skills, and need support in doing so. Specialist colleges like Foxes do a huge amount of work in helping such young people to take control of their lives – particularly in the residential sense, where living away from home in a group provides both a degree of independence and preparation for a life beyond the family home. This is, after all, the norm for most university students, in halls of residence and shared houses.

There are about 70 specialist further education colleges in the UK, most offering residential care, but places can cost more than £30,000 a year, and for students with complex needs over £150,000. Many young people and their families face a long battle to secure funding, particularly (as is often the case) when the one that best serves their needs is in another local authority. Sarah and her friends do not want to be reliant on benefits and wish, like everyone else, to be given the chance to prove themselves in the workplace. Specialist colleges improve the outcomes and quality of life for students with complex needs, and give them confidence in the key area of employment.

Foxes Academy has achieved an Ofsted grade 1 'outstanding' rating, and since its inception has successfully seen hundreds of young people with learning disabilities graduate. Over 86 per cent of learners from the past five years have found employment after leaving, and about 75 per cent are living semi-independently. The Academy now has ten residential houses in Minehead, and at any one time around 80 learners. It also offers short-stay respite breaks and holidays for young people aged over 16.

In 2015 Channel 5 broadcast a television documentary series about Foxes, *The Special Needs Hotel*. Sarah had left by then, but the show featured some of her friends and many of her beloved staff members. The series proved popular viewing and was received with great acclaim, though, unbelievably, there was still someone who set up a spoof site on Facebook which not only slated the show but uploaded some shockingly offensive images, including one of a small child with Down's syndrome drowning in a washing machine. Foxes reported the abuse, as did a number of parents, but Facebook's response was that it didn't breach their guidelines before it was finally removed. Avon and Somerset Police were also informed, but no action was taken. Yet another instance of the abuse of the learning-disabled apparently being acceptable.

Sarah graduated in July 2014 and achieved a Level 1 NVQ in Food and Beverage Service, and Level 1 award in Food Safety – neither of which was adapted in any way for people with learning disabilities. All the family travelled down to Minehead for the big day, which was a huge celebration of all the learners' achievements. But even more exciting for all of us was that, much to her surprise, Sarah was awarded the prize of being the year's outstanding student, and received a cup, which was duly added to her silverware cupboard.

Sarah was naturally thrilled, and we couldn't help but compare her ecstatic feelings with the forlorn mood when we had left her that first day at Foxes nearly three years previously.

In July 2017 Sarah was asked back to Foxes to be guest speaker at their graduation ceremony. We travelled down to Minehead and stayed in the hotel again, and Sarah was suitably emotional, showing me her old haunts. The trip brought back all the happy times she'd had there, and a few tears were shed. We met many of the staff who had helped Sarah, and she was greeted like a homecoming queen. The celebrated TV chef Brian Turner CBE was the guest of honour and, clearly touched by the occasion and the pride of the students in their achievements, gave a very emotional speech. Sarah was nervous, but delivered the speech we'd written together beautifully, even timing the jokes to perfection – her grandfather would have been proud. Here's an extract.

> Hi, I'm Sarah and I'm 25. It's great to be back at Foxes where I spent three happy years until I graduated in 2014 ... all the learners and house managers and staff were brilliant. They were all caring and kind and taught me a lot. Like all of you I did housekeeping and food preparation, but my favourite was food service and I always wanted to do that for a job.
>
> I had a wonderful experience at Foxes and loved every minute. . . I'd like to thank everyone here for

their help and giving me all these opportunities. And a special mention for Ben Graham who is amazing! Congratulations to everyone who has graduated and good luck in your careers in hospitality and catering! I'm sure that going to Foxes will help all of you.

Have a wonderful day and a wonderful life!

Ben Graham, who manages Work Experience and Transition at Foxes and was awarded an MBE in 2017 for his work with young adults with learning disabilities, emailed me afterwards.

Several people commented afterwards how well she spoke, and how her talk inspired others to similarly go into the world with skills, confidence and a passion to succeed as Sarah has. She truly is an amazing ambassador for Foxes, and like yourselves we are truly very proud of her.

We travelled back to London on the train with Brian Turner and his lovely manager Louise, but had to stand most of the way from Taunton due to an earlier derailment which resulted in hundreds of extra passengers on board. In fact, there was even barely room to stand, and Sarah gave up the seat we'd reserved as we found it already occupied, coincidentally, by a young Scandinavian child with DS, who was exhausted and needed to sleep.

A couple of weeks later a message from a Kirstie Edwards was posted on the Foxes Facebook page.

Hi there! I met a really wonderful young woman called Sarah in a train to London on Friday . . . she was truly a credit to herself firstly, but also to the training and support you must have provided...I was a rather fed-up, emotional traveller with arthritis, and we had a life-affirming chat. We experience the opposite sides of the same coin – I am disabled, but no-one can see it, so people over-estimate and question me, and she is disabled, and people under-estimate and undervalue her worth. She proudly told me how lucky she is – as am I. Anyway, I just wanted to tell her how lovely it was to meet her, and thank her for being understanding when I was upset. What a lovely woman.

13

SILENTLY CLOSING
HER BEDROOM DOOR

However painful the process of leaving home, for parents and for children, the really frightening thing for both would be the prospect of the child never leaving home.

Robert Neelly Bellah

A Jewish man goes to a psychiatrist, and immediately launches into his problem. 'Oh, doctor, I can't sleep, I can't eat – I'm a wreck. You see, every time I fall asleep I have these terrible, vivid dreams, and in these dreams my mother is everywhere. She is everywhere!'

'Now, I can see this is a problem,' the shrink begins to explain, 'but –'

'No, you don't understand,' the man interrupts. 'It's not just that. In my dreams I meet other people, completely different people – and then they all turn into my mother! Everyone turns into my mother! And I toss and turn all night, and when I wake up I'm covered in sweat. I tell you, it's all I can do to stagger downstairs in the morning and make myself a coffee and a piece of toast.'

The psychiatrist shakes his head sadly, and then says, 'What? One piece of toast for a big boy like you?'

Silently Closing Her Bedroom Door

Allie has never played the role of the classic Jewish mother. In fact, we were always clear that we wanted Sarah to be independent of us in the same way as Daniel and Joel, and in order to be able to achieve this, finding suitable accommodation was going to be vital. This was something we had first envisaged for Sarah when she was, to paraphrase A. A. Milne, only 'one and had just begun'. As tempting as it would be to keep Sarah safe by continuing to have her live with us, this would inevitably prevent her from leading her own, individual life. There is a fine balance between protection and stifling. And, an even greater worry, we had always been concerned about would happen to her when we were no longer around. Her brothers would always be there to love and support her, but there shouldn't be an expectation that in the future Sarah would live with either of them and their partners.

As I wrote in *A Minor Adjustment*,

> Once she is an adult, we will encourage her to move to whatever type of housing is most suitable. We hope that Sarah might be able to manage a flat of her own, or a place that she could share with friends. Although I would obviously prefer to see Sarah completely integrated, this sort of provision does at least provide security and stability in a semi-independent setting, where she would have the opportunity to make a positive contribution to a community.

The most worrying scenario would have been if Sarah hadn't been capable of living even in a semi-independent setting, and had to live in an institution. There's the further concern about abuse in some of these establishments, which is still occurring much too frequently.

When Sarah left Foxes, the staff were quite clear that she should not return home for any length of time before moving to accommodation beyond the clutches of her family:

> Sarah needs to have accommodation and occupation in place when she leaves. Any delay will also lead to an erosion of the extensive independent-living and employment skills that she has worked so hard for during her time at Foxes Academy. She must be given the support and every opportunity to make a positive contribution to society and to lead a fulfilling life.

We had started considering options at the end of Sarah's second year in Minehead, but there didn't seem a great deal of choice. There was one residential community in north London that seemed a possibility, although at first we weren't sure that the Langdon Community, a Jewish charity for adults with learning difficulties, would be the right choice: I'm not Jewish and Allie isn't religious. However, Allie did know of the charity through her work, and had always heard positive things.

An appointment was made for a social worker from the Langdon to visit. When we told Sarah that someone called Simone was coming to meet us, she said this must be the Simone who had taught her sex education at the sixth-form centre in Haringey.

'No, Sarah,' we told her, 'this can't be that Simone. This is a completely different organisation. You've definitely got it wrong.'

Of course, Sarah had got it right . . . as usual.

As soon as Simone arrived, she and Sarah greeted each other like long-lost sisters and Simone's warmth and professionalism, and her description of life at the Community, convinced us that the Langdon and Sarah were absolutely right for each other. My only concern was that Simone later told us Sarah had been the star pupil in her sex education class – not something a dad needs to know.

We talked about Sarah's support needs, which was four hours of daily care, to include help with personal hygiene, preparing meals, shopping, cleaning, budgeting and travel training. We also felt that in the early days Sarah would need a lot of reassurance and support from Langdon staff, as change didn't always come that easily to her and she did sometimes become flustered in new situations. This was clearly a life-changing move, but we had faith that, as in the past, with time and good support she would adjust.

There was no waiting list, as Langdon rented property in the area as and when according to need, and thus Allie, Sarah and I visited her proposed accommodation in north London about half an hour's drive from us. The house, close to shops and public transport links, was modern and fresh, with a lovely warm atmosphere and, most importantly, without a hint of being institutional. We were immediately convinced that Sarah would thrive in this welcoming home, which she would share with three other residents and staff members. The available room was perfect, and made more so when it was agreed it could be re-decorated and painted in Sarah's favourite shade of 'sexy pink'. This was a place she could call her own home, and where, most importantly, she could stay forever.

We can recall so clearly the weight being lifted from our shoulders. All my fears for the future were allayed, and when I imagined Sarah in her cosy attic space, living her own life and making her own choices, I was reduced to tears. Not just a tear in the eye, not simply a trickle. I have to admit I blubbed.

Funding was duly agreed with Haringey Council for the

Langdon fees, and a date was set for her move. Sarah was thrilled and, in preparation, went on a trip to Henley to meet some of the other members of the Community. She spent two nights there, and then moved in to her new north London home on the last day of August 2014. A 'welcome buffet' was arranged for her, to which the whole family were invited. 'When we dropped Sarah off at Langdon it felt like it was for good,' wrote Daniel later, 'and as I listened to "She's Leaving Home" on the way back to Mum and Dad's I felt particularly choked as I realised that she had managed to move out before me.'

Sarah did miss Foxes initially, and later accused of us moving her to Langdon too quickly, as she would have liked to spend more time with us at home before moving on, but we're still not sure why she holds these views, as she settled in to her new home with very little fuss. She was greatly helped by her then house manager, Vicky, and soon had a plethora of activities to occupy her, in which she met other members of the community who lived in various flats and houses in the local area.

Sarah made lots of friends very quickly, and flourished amid all the social aspects of Langdon like yoga, coffee evenings, pub trips, Shabbat dinners, regular parties and outings and going to the gym. She also volunteered in a charity shop and undertook some duties at the Langdon's reception.

As I write, Sarah has been at Langdon three years, where she is secure, happy and stimulated, supported by a team of devoted, skilled and hard-working support workers. This is her verdict.

> I really feel part of the Langdon community. I love my house and my house mates, Leah, Gabby and Tanya are brilliant. My support workers are lovely and really helpful too if I have a problem. My manager, 'Mags'

teaches me not to stress and I really can talk to her. Sophie is her daughter and we have lots of fun. great. Demi takes me swimming and there is Nicola, who is a brilliant chef, I have lots of chats with Jolanta – she makes me laugh all the time. Flower (Elizabeth) is amazing – very helpful to me. I interviewed Patsy, who is now my keyworker and she is great.

As you may have gathered, I can't imagine Sarah being happier anywhere else.

14

KITCHEN IMPOSSIBLE

Ask not what you can do for your country.
Ask what's for lunch.

Orson Welles

As I have said earlier, I'm not terribly happy about the stereotypes associated with Down's syndrome – I don't like using 'they' as a describe-all for people with DS. 'They' are individuals and every one is unique, but sometimes you can't help but put your hands up and admit defeat.

The love of food is an absolute, and matched only by the addiction to soap operas. Probably up north *Coronation Street* rules supreme, but down south Sarah and all her friends love *EastEnders*. Boy bands and girl groups also feature heavily. In fact, a blood test may not be necessary to ascertain the condition: medics should just wait until 'they' are in their teens and inquire as to whether they like Westlife, the Spice Girls and *EastEnders* – no spilling of blood would be required, and you'd have a 100 per cent accurate answer.

There was a wonderful moment at a Shifting Perspectives exhibition on the South Bank when word got out that *EastEnders* actor Perry Fenwick was in the room. A group of young adults dashed towards the back of the room where Perry was looking at the photographs, but they had to pass a buffet table laden with goodies, and so came to a sudden stop. A terrible dilemma, which was resolved by a quick raid of the *canapés* and continuation of the sprint to hug Perry.

Like Damon Runyon's character Nicely Nicely Johnson, Sarah is dearly 'committed to eating', and much of her waking life revolves around food and discussion of the next repast. She once famously said, while tucking in to afternoon tea, 'My chocolate cake is addicted to me.' When we used to tell her that we were 'just making do' for dinner, the expression on her face could be compared to the subject of Munch's 'The Scream'. Coupled with her sixth-form studies and three years at Foxes, it was somewhat inevitable that future employment would be gravy-based. Quite how, we weren't sure, but again providence played a part.

In March 2015, Sarah became involved in a project that has changed her life immeasurably. Her friend Annalie, whom Sarah has known since babyhood, was asked to take part in a four-part reality television series on Channel 4 in which the participants, a group of eight adults with learning disabilities, would be mentored by the chef Michel Roux Jr and his staff with a view to finding them jobs in the catering and hospitality profession. Michel Roux Jr spoke about the series with enthusiasm: 'I am passionate about the restaurant industry, and in my mind there should be no barrier to work. I'm thrilled to be part of a project that celebrates people's abilities, challenges perceptions and hopefully transforms lives.' He admitted the industry is not the best for employing people with disabilities. 'There is a huge pool of talent out there . . . too often people can be written off. In my experience, everyone has potential. It's just a matter of giving them that chance to prove it.'

A Major Adjustment

The producers were looking for other contributors, and good old Annalie suggested her mate Sarah. With the support of Michel's charity Springboard, which helps disadvantaged young people into the hospitality industry, the series would follow the participants as they were trained and undertook work experience, and then attempts would be made to secure employment for them.

Sarah was incredibly fortunate to be chosen, because the production company, Twofour Wales, had interviewed hundreds of candidates. Allie and I wanted to be certain that the show was legit, and that Twofour was a responsible company, and so we did some background research. In fact, they proved to be totally professional at every level, and we were convinced they would act in Sarah's interests, although we knew that, being television, entertainment would be their priority.

While we were obviously pleased for Sarah, we also wanted her to be sure this was something she really wanted to do. Sarah and I met with the company's psychologist, therefore, who questioned her about how she might cope with being in the spotlight, and handle any publicity, and how she would react if she was recognised and approached. There was also the possibility of internet bullying and trolling. We made sure Sarah wouldn't post anything about the show, and the producers promised support throughout.

The group would also live together for short periods of time while filming and training (some of the time in a secluded house in the Surrey countryside, otherwise in a Hackney flat), and Twofour appointed three chaperones who would be responsible for both their safeguarding during the filming and any 'pastoral' care. One of the chaperones, Guy Milnes, is also a professional photographer who has worked regularly on various TV and film projects, as well as a carer, and later became a manager at the

Kitchen Impossible

National Centre for Young People with Epilepsy. 'Nothing could quite prepare me for what lay ahead over four weeks,' he later wrote of his experience on the series.

> I can say that my time on *Kitchen Impossible* was one of my most beautiful and worthwhile experiences. Working so closely with the eight contributors, we quickly became very fond of them. I think it was a huge learning curve for all involved, and the production team were keen to listen to us and work together for the good of the trainees.

Allie and I completed a questionnaire assessing Sarah's personal needs, and the answers we gave do highlight Sarah's capabilities at the time:

> Because of Sarah's learning disability she does longer to understand instructions and needs repetitive guidance.

> Because of her Down's syndrome she is physically slower than able-bodied adults.

> She is very sociable and polite, and has had quite a lot of experience greeting guests and waiting on tables at the Foxes hotel, and on work experience working in a college café.

> Sarah is very good with simple tasks – anything new, slightly complicated or abstract might hinder her, and she would need some supervision.

Sarah might need to be explained anything new a few times, and often says she understands when she doesn't really grasp what is required. She sometimes becomes flustered if she doesn't know exactly what to do. Once a new element is learned she is fine.

We think Sarah would find it difficult to work under pressure in a very busy kitchen. She will be much better 'front of house' or waitressing, if supervised. Just reassurance, an arm around the shoulder, boosting her confidence.

She soon comes around, and doesn't sulk or stay upset for very long. You know where you stand with Sarah – she will show or tell you exactly what she is feeling.

It was at this time, in April 2015, that Clare Walsh from Foxes Academy first wrote to us, asking if Sarah would like to be guest speaker at their annual graduation. I had to respond that Sarah would have loved to be part of the event, but was filming a television series! When Sarah was born those were words I never thought I'd find myself saying.

Filming for the series began, and I travelled with Sarah and Annalie's mother Michelle to the Orpington campus of Bromley College, where Sarah met Michel and his team (Abby and Rob) and the other participants. While being filmed, each of them had to prepare a 'signature dish', and we decided scrambled eggs with chorizo and some asparagus was a fairly safe option for Sarah, although she didn't have time to practise and, on tasting, Michel described her dish as 'a bit dry.'

Sarah was immediately apologetic. 'Oh, sorry, Michel!'

Kitchen Impossible

Jack, who has autism and worked in the kitchen of a Hertfordshire pub ('I'm probably the best kitchen porter in the world'), captured everyone's hearts by re-heating a prepared chicken tikka masala meal in the microwave – 'Should be absolutely delicious' –and then referring to his mentor as 'the sexy, handsome Michel Rouge'.

There was an immediate bond between Sam and Sophie – both were 17 and, having Tourette's syndrome, prone to some colourful language. Sophie disarmingly described her condition as 'like having a naughty child in your brain telling you to do this . . . do this . . . do this.' She had applied for 170 jobs, but had only got two interviews. She also stated that her 'ticks' disappeared when she was cooking, but that morning suffered a severe attack which left Michel shaken. 'I'd never seen Tourette's syndrome manifest itself like that before with those physical ticks.'

The other participants were Ben, 30, a charming Yorkshire lad who has Asperger's, Beth, 23, who was born with Apert syndrome, and Dan, 24, a chef who a few months earlier had been cooking at an army barracks until complications arising out of diabetes led to him to losing his sight. 'When I went blind the Jobcentre told me I might as well tear up my CV and start again, but I don't know what else I can do. I love the heat of the kitchen.'

The following day, the group travelled to Hawksmoor restaurant in Knightsbridge to help with the lunchtime shift. This would give them an understanding of 'real work' and make them appreciate the high standard that would be expected of them in the following weeks. While Sarah worked in the kitchen, Annalie was waitressing. In a lovely moment, Annalie was juggling a couple of plates on a tray and an expensive sirloin steak dropped on to her chest. Without hesitation, she returned it to the plate and served it to a surprised but extremely tolerant diner.

A Major Adjustment

The following day Allie and I, along with members of the other contributors' families and a number of chefs, were invited to lunch at the college. Michel soon concluded that Sarah's skills were more suited to front of house than in the kitchen, and so she performed a waitressing role. She was so professional she made no eye contact with us! She helped served up a delicious meal of Sushi Canapés, Soufflé Suisse, and Saddle of Hogget, stuffed with creamed spinach and spices, followed by Lemon Tart with a White Chocolate Sorbet and Bitter Orange Sauce. The soufflé was created by Michel's father, the world-renowned chef Albert Roux, in the 1960s, and was now one of Michel's signature dishes.

Unfortunately, the soufflés proved to be temperamental and, while being filmed by half a dozen camera crews, some of the guests had to wait quite a long time to be served. Allie and I didn't wish to be critical and were very patient, although I think the crew were hoping we would be a bit more stroppy to make for better television. There was an incredibly emotional moment when chef Dan, who was responsible for the saddle of hogget, was led out by Michel and announced his dish to the luncheon guests. At the end of the meal all eight participants came out to meet us, and Michel gave a little speech: 'There were errors, and we have a long way to go. But hopefully they are proud of what they have achieved. So much to learn, but they can learn anything.'

An incident in the second episode showed how seriously Michel was taking his role of mentor. The group was preparing lunch for members of the public at Bromley College, but all the prawns for the main dish were left unrefrigerated, and because of the health risk could not be served. Sam, appointed as head chef, felt responsible, and the mistake brought her to tears. Michel was clearly angry – and gave all the participants a proper ticking-off. All the gang were clearly disappointed, but no-one individual was held responsible: they shouldered the blame as a team, and a valuable lesson was learned.

They recovered themselves brilliantly a few days later by achieving success at Michel's pop-up restaurant at the Taste of London food festival in Regent's Park. He designed a menu that enabled his trainees to demonstrate how much they had already learnt. Their dishes were hugely popular, and they coped with long queues. Michel had entrusted Sam in the role of head chef again, and this time he sailed through with flying colours.

Sarah then gained some work experience at Fratelli La Bufala, an Italian restaurant on Shaftesbury Avenue. The manager, Enzo, was great with Sarah, and she thoroughly enjoyed her time there. We did go there for dinner *en famille* one evening before going to see *Guys and Dolls*, and we were given very special treatment.

The third episode ended with the team preparing and serving a meal at Roux at Parliament Square, one of Michel's restaurants. Beth, normally shy and self-conscious, was in the kitchen and shouting out orders 'running the pass'. Initially reticent at having to be so bossy, by the end she was barking out orders. 'Very moving – I've shouted like I've never shouted. I never thought I could do it.'

We had been sent the third episode prior to the broadcast, and I was a bit concerned that Sarah had been featured very little either in this one or the other episodes. I didn't care that all the filming that had been done with me and the rest of the family was edited out (although the bit where we were filmed in our own kitchen producing an almost inedible pasta dish, with Allie dropping a rusty saucepan handle into the pasta sauce, might have provided some comic relief), but there hadn't been one interview with Sarah on her own, and the viewer wouldn't have known anything about her.

A Major Adjustment

I rang the executive producer, Sam Grace. Having been raised in the world of entertainment and television, I knew only too well how the medium worked. The trouble was that Sarah just got on with the job, didn't cause a fuss, and so didn't make for dramatic television. Sam was apologetic, but I just wanted to make sure that Sarah had a bit of a part in the final episode. Sarah herself was unconcerned, but the same was true of the charming and capable Ben, who had barely been seen so far, and was upset. But that is the nature of the beast, and the participants were warned beforehand, 'You might find that you are featured more than other contributors, or you might be featured less.'

The final episode featured a reception for potential employers, when 85 representatives of restaurants and hotels were invited to an event to meet the contributors – a sort of job fair. The group prepared and served canapés, and job interviews followed, when the trainees were advised by Michel to have 'nerves of steel'.

Then, a fabulous, morale-boosting trip to Paris, in which the group organised a dinner for seven members of Michel's family, after procuring the provisions for a classic French menu at a local market. Their biggest critic initially was Albert Roux, Michel's father – 'I'm not fussy: I simply I know what I like.' But then he was full of praise for the Millefeuille – 'Better than some restaurants' – and ended up by pronouncing it 'a wonderful meal.' He was clearly moved by the whole event, and it ended with him kissing Michel: 'Good job, I'm proud of you.' It was very touching.

The dénouement charted the future careers of the participants. Jack, although a great character and perfect for front of house, didn't want to give up his dishwashing job, as he felt comfortable in his role and enjoyed the work. Sam and Sophie both got employed as chefs, and had become involved romantically, much to the excitement of Sarah and Annalie, who were delighted for them. Beth gained employment as a waitress in a café, and Ben was employed as a food and beverage operative in a hotel. Annalie was employed as front-of-house in a sushi restaurant, but Dan needed time to come to terms with the recent loss of his sight, and decided to attend a specialist college for the blind.

Sarah was finally featured on her own in the show when she received a telephone call at home from Kevin, the manager of the Thistle Hotel in Bayswater, offering her a job. She obviously knew the call was coming, but genuinely didn't know what he was going to say. Initially she was excited and shocked at the news – 'I've got it!' Then she broke down in tears, and through her crying managed to say, 'I'm really happy!'

Although we would have loved to see more of Sarah, the most important thing was how so sensitively the participants were depicted – without being patronised. 'With voices seldom heard on TV, it's a cut above standard fussing about sautés', ran the *Guardian*'s review, praising Michel Roux Jr for his mentoring role in tutoring protégés in a firm, unpatronising way, despite admitting there were moments when he wondered what on earth he'd taken on:

> All our contributors were challenged in a major way. We didn't want them to fail, but if they did, it was about drawing out the positives, so they could learn for next time. . . It's been emotional. You want to hug them and cajole, but that's doing them a disservice.

Kitchen Impossible was a very positive portrayal of the disability world we have inhabited for over 25 years, and was touching, entertaining and educative. There was a genuine rapport and support among the participants. Twofour didn't put a foot wrong throughout the whole process – Sarah's welfare was paramount, and all our queries were answered immediately. The organisation was incredibly efficient, and every single member of the talented team we met or spoke to was helpful and understanding. Sarah had the most fantastic time, and still speaks fondly of all the friends she made.

In May 2016, Sarah and I were asked to address 550 guests at a Langdon charity dinner event held at Wembley Stadium. Accompanied by his charming wife Giselle, the guest of honour was Michel. We were to follow him onto the platform, but when Sarah saw how many people there were in the room, the huge screens on which she would be featured, and the enormity of the occasion, she had a slight meltdown and became tearful. She didn't think she could go on. I told her not to worry, and said I would read her speech for her. But she gathered herself and, after Michel's heartfelt and inspiring speech, and a montage of clips from the show, Sarah strode on to the platform by my side and, once centre-stage, there was no stopping her. Ad-libbing, playing to the crowd, interrupting my 'bon mots', like the several generations of ancestral performers in the family she was an absolute trouper.

She thanked Michel for the experience, and apologised to him for a scene in the series in which she had mangled some asparagus tips. The incident, now known in the family as Asparagusgate, has become family folklore, and when Sarah needs taking down a peg or two we speak of little else.

The following day she sent me a text, which simply read, 'We smashed it.'

15

THE DIGNITY OF LABOUR

Find a job you enjoy doing, and you will never have to work a day in your life.

Mark Twain

Being at work doesn't just mean being able to have money for decent housing and standard of living: it also provides you with choices about lifestyle and the pursuit of leisure activities, and means feeling valued, while at the same time contributing to society. The workplace is where you make friends, where you can realise some of your aspirations and where, most importantly, people with learning disabilities can feel independent.

But if finding employment is hard enough for most job seekers, it's particularly challenging for someone with Down's syndrome. Although many people with Down's are more than capable of holding down a variety of jobs, the odds are stacked against them being employed, for reasons that have nothing to do with their abilities or commitment. People with disabilities are four times more likely to be unemployed, and the employment rate of adults with learning disabilities is less than six per cent – we are one of the few European countries without legislation to enforce companies to employ people with disabilities.

Sarah has been very lucky, because without the advantage of

appearing on *Kitchen Impossible*, and the contacts and links that Michel Roux Jr was able to provide, it's very unlikely that she would have landed such suitable employment. Soon after she was offered the job at one of the Thistle hotels, my first concern was that behind it might be a disingenuous attempt to attract positive publicity in front of millions of television viewers. I wondered how sincere the offer of work really was and whether, once Sarah was out of the television spotlight, the hoteliers might decide she wasn't quite what they were looking for. So I arranged a meeting with Sarah and her future managers.

Both Kevin Gonsalves, who had delivered the good news to Sarah on the telephone during the filming, and the hotel's general manager Andrew Byrne were keen to meet. They listened to my concerns, and I was immediately put at ease by their response. Andrew repeated something he had said on the show. 'We have certain expectations that everybody that works for us delivers to the standards we expect. We are a big chain,' he added, 'and don't need to employ Sarah for publicity purposes. We saw her in action at the reception and were impressed by her.' I in turn assured them that I wouldn't be checking up on her at every turn, and hovering around the hotel for the first sign of any possible exploitation of my girl.

Following some travel training, Sarah learned a couple of London Underground routes from her home to work, and soon mastered her Tube commute. Her job description was that of a 'food and beverage operative', and her main tasks would be to meet and greet guests before showing them to the breakfast table, lay and clear tables, and respond to any queries about the breakfast buffet. Sarah started work at the hotel in October 2015 for three mornings a week, providing breakfast service. Her starting time was 8 a.m., but she would often be there an hour early!

The Dignity Of Labour

Sandor Megyeri, Sarah's present manager has been incredibly supportive.

> By working with Sarah we have learnt a lot, and as a result have adapted our working environment to provide her with the support she needs. She shows us that people with disabilities can provide the same quality, and can give a bit extra in customer service by being completely genuine and giving 100 per cent all the time. I truly believe by working with Sarah I became a proper manager, as I have adapted the knowledge to treat everyone on the same level.

What I found shocking was that Sarah was the first person with a disability that Sandor had worked with, even though he has been working in the hotel trade in London's West End for over a decade. But again, the synchronicity that has underpinned Sarah's life continued to work its magic, as Sandor's wife works with children with special needs, and so he had some understanding of Down's. Sarah has been wholeheartedly accepted by her work mates as part of the hard-working team, and this was typified when she attended Kevin Gonsalves' leaving do. I had to accompany Sarah, and met most of her colleagues, who mainly hailed from eastern and central Europe, and was so touched to see how they related to her, and how valued and respected she was as part of their close-knit team.

In October 2016, Sarah was invited to attend a round-table meeting at the Department of Education, as part of Work Experience Week, in which representatives from various organisations discussed the opportunities – or lack of them – for people with learning disabilities to gain employment. The conference was run by Fair Train, an institution, which provides coaching, information, advice and guidance to employers and learners on all forms of work experience. Employers, employees, colleges and policy makers reported their situation, and the initiatives they had in place to increase and improve opportunities. Sarah herself described the difference having a job made in all aspects of her life, made relevant contributions and 'informed' a representative of the Department of Education.

There has always been much evidence that people with learning disabilities make excellent employees, as they tend to stay in the job for longer than their non-disabled colleagues, exhibit a strong commitment to work, are punctual and have low rates of absenteeism. Not only can they make a positive impact across the workforce but, in addition, the public think more highly of companies that employ disabled people.

The challenge is to spread the word, and make it the norm for all employers to be positive about employing disabled people, as it appears too many haven't yet realised the genuine commercial benefits. Over seven million people of working age (17.5 per cent) in the UK are disabled or have a health condition – a lot of talent that companies are missing out on. Despite strategies over many years, and innovative work by employers, colleges, training providers and the voluntary sector, sustainable employment opportunities for significant numbers of disabled people have remained pitifully low.

During Work Experience Week, colleges and employers signed up to being Disability Confident, a voluntary DWP (Department of Work and Pensions) scheme aimed at helping employers make the most of the opportunities provided by employing disabled people. It is somewhat ironic that, following this conference, the DWP used Sarah as their 'poster girl' on their social media outlets, although her gainful employment had nothing to do with their efforts.

Ten years ago, the Down's Syndrome Association launched a telling and somewhat pointed poignant poster campaign, using a picture of a young man with Down's, with the strapline, 'You've now been looking at Paul longer than any employer ever has.' The charity's 'WorkFit' programme has been running since 2011, and provides advice on how employees can best support a work colleague with the condition. It stresses the importance of having the right support network in the early stages of work, developing a job plan, the importance of a mentor or workplace ally, and colleagues having an awareness about the condition, which can better enable them to provide the necessary help.

Since 2011, 182 candidates have been in placed in various meaningful jobs as a result of the campaign. Of the 182 placed, 100 people are in permanent paid work, and among the sectors in which adults with DS have been placed are the public sector, tourism, construction, catering, retail and finance. Obviously this is only one scheme, the numbers are relatively small and, because of the lack of employment opportunities, some parents who are in a position to do so have actually set up their own business, particularly in catering.

Tim's Place is an eatery in Albuquerque, New Mexico owned by Tim Harris, a young man with Down's. As far as I know it is the only restaurant in the world owned by a person with the syndrome, and was set up by his parents in 2010. The restaurant places an emphasis on friendliness, and Tim serves customers with 'plenty of hugs' alongside their huevos rancheros and green chile burgers. In Illinois, Nancy Gianni founded a charity GiGi's Playhouse to promote 'awareness and community acceptance' following the birth of her daughter GiGi in 2004, and recently opened a café, Hugs and Mugs (yes, yet more hugs), which is staffed entirely by people with Down's syndrome, or Down syndrome as it is referred to Stateside and in certain quarters this side of the pond. Allie and I visited a similar establishment in the Netherlands. More locally, in north London, a group called WAVE (We Are All Valued Equally) runs a pop-up café with a view to setting up a permanent establishment.

I had met the businesswoman Rosa Monckton some years previously at the demonstration in support of specialist colleges (see chapter 12). Her daughter Domenica, who was born in 1995, has Down's and, being influenced by her aunt, Nigella Lawson, studied catering at Brighton City College. Rosa was frustrated by the problems Domenica faced when in terms of statutory responsibility she became an adult:

> Once a child finishes full-time education, everything shuts down. Nothing has changed just because, in the eyes of the law, they have become adults overnight: they have the rest of their lives ahead of them. Trying to ensure that Domenica is fully part of a community – in the sense of being actively a part of the world, whether that be at school, college or work – became all consuming . . . work is vital for personal growth and a sense of self-worth. Even if someone is only capable of doing a few hours a week, the sense of self-esteem and belonging that comes from being part of a team is invaluable.

Rosa Monckton's idea was to launch a course in supported employment for young adults, and so she started Team Domenica, a Brighton-based charity, to meets the needs of learning-disabled young adults whose greatest challenge is to find regular employment. The charity has a training centre and café and an employment agency: 'Through this we provide employment programmes set up to help prepare candidates for the workplace, access employment, make new friends, and feel better connected to their local community.' The aim is to become a national charity, starting with another four centres to be opened in the next three years.

Rosa is a fantastic advocate for Down's syndrome and learning disability, and in 2017 was recognised for her commitment to the cause with the award of an MBE. There is one area, however, in which I take issue with her. In 2017, she wrote an article in the *Spectator* arguing that learning-disabled people should be allowed to work for a lower hourly rate than the minimum wage. 'A therapeutic exemption from the minimum wage would have a transformative effect,' she wrote. 'The single thing that makes it most difficult to get people with learning disabilities into work is the ratcheting up of the minimum wage.'

I strongly believe that receiving the same salary helps employees to feel valued the same as their co-workers, and treated as equal citizens. A differential in wages could also legitimise the assumption that people with learning disabilities might not do their job properly, and thus should be paid less. 'There is no evidence that minimum wage is pricing people out of work,' the chief executive of the National Development Team for Inclusion, Rob Greig, has written.

> People with learning disabilities are out of work because of a combination of negative attitudes and not having access to the right support. People are not out of work because of pay levels: they are out of work because they are not getting the right support . . .

> working for less money is not a route into long-term
> paid work.

And in December 2017, the prospect of more people with disabilities being employed was hardly enhanced by a statement from the Chancellor of the Exchequer. Asked by the Treasury Select Committee about the sluggish economic growth Philip Hammond replied, 'It is almost certainly the case that by increasing participation in the workforce, including far higher levels of participation by marginal groups and very high levels of engagement in the workforce, for example of disabled people – something we should be extremely proud of – [this] may have had an impact on overall productivity measurements.'

Since Sarah started earning she has a better grasp of budgeting, and the value of money in general. In fact, she used to be much more generous, and, now that she appreciates the value of her labour, has become a little more parsimonious!

I happened to be passing Sarah's hotel some months ago with Maureen, a friend visiting from the USA. I mentioned that Sarah was at work that day, and so we thought we would pop in and say hello. We strode in thinking she would be happy to see us. Breakfast service had finished, the guests had all gone, and it seemed a perfect time.

Sarah's face was thunderous. Instead of the usual kiss, cuddle and warm greeting, she said somewhat frostily, 'What are you doing here?'

I told her that we had really wanted to see her and say hi. Those words buttered no parsnips.

'I'm working. You should have let me know.'

I explained that it was a spontaneous decision, and Maureen wanted to see where she worked.

'You still should have let me know,' was again the response.

One of her colleagues told Sarah it was fine to join us, as the restaurant was now very quiet, sat us down and went off to get us a couple of coffees. Sarah reluctantly joined us, but it was obvious she was uncomfortable and, for what must have been the first time in her life, didn't want to socialise. She was still at work, and had various duties to perform before she finished her shift. I quickly realised that she wasn't going to be happy sitting with us, and suggested she return to her work. Relieved, Sarah got up and was about to speak, but before she could say anything, I interrupted. 'I know. "You should have told me. . ."'

At first, I'd been a bit miffed at the rebuff, but I could now see it from Sarah's point of view. We had disturbed her at work, and most people wouldn't necessarily be pleased about that. She had acted in a completely professional way, and both Maureen and I were proud of her.

Daniel had also been to see Sarah at the hotel, but he'd the wherewithal to forewarn her.

> For Sarah, food is a serious business, and she is a serious professional. What is great is that Sarah's job revolves around one of her main passions, which is not something many can say. I've loved watching her in action on the odd time she's let me crash her breakfast service at the hotel with friends as non-hotel guests. I wasn't at all surprised seeing her in action for the first time – it's what she'd wanted for so long, and she leapt at the chance. She's a stickler, and I'm proud that her skills and a commitment to quality service have been recognised, even if it took a TV programme to fast-track her to a plush London hotel.

A Major Adjustment

Sarah has now been in her job for over two years, attends staff meetings, has worked at one of the other Thistle hotels, and is training as a barista. She is carving out a career for herself – something we never would have believed could have happened.

'Sarah is a great asset to the business,' wrote Richard O'Riordan, Thistle Hotels' General Manager recently. 'Her enthusiasm to engage with customers and colleagues is admirable. She is confident, professional, and has a positive outlook that is infectious. Sarah is now an important part of our successful team and a joy to work with.'

I'm looking forward to seeing Sarah at work again in the near future, comfortable in her role and performing her duties with charm and skill. But next time I'll give her 28 days' notice, in writing.

16

A LEVEL PLAYING FIELD

Let me win, but if I cannot win, let me be brave in the attempt.

Special Olympics credo

Sport has always played an important part in our family's life. Rightly or wrongly, we aren't far behind Bill Shankly, when he was asked, 'Do you think football is a matter of life and death?' and replied, 'Oh, no, it's much more important than that.'

There was a time when Sarah was just as keen on football as her brothers, and used to play with them in the local park, or even in our hallway. During a World Cup qualifying match against Italy, Daniel was singing the words to 'Three Lions – Football's Coming Home' and, with her usual mixture of sociability and inquisitiveness, Sarah looked up and said, 'To my house?'

Sadly, Sarah's football career ended at Foxes Academy, when she felt aggrieved that one of her friends seemed to be taking all the corners and, in a fit of pique, decided to hang up her boots. Fortunately, she still enjoys the sport as a spectator, and loves going to the Spurs, where mood swings from 'sick as a parrot' to 'over the moon' can be gauged by Tottenham's result.

The national game, which in the past never provided the opportunity for learning-disabled players to participate, is now much more geared up to inclusivity. In 2004, the first Down's syndrome football team, the Fulham Badgers, was formed, in partnership between the DSA and Fulham FC's Community Sports Trust, its charitable arm. Two years later, a Down's Syndrome Football Festival was held at Motspur Park, Fulham's training ground, in which nine teams and eighty-four players participated. Not only did the players have the chance to take part in what was for many of them their first competitive football tournament, but the day also provided an ideal opportunity for disability coaches from all over the country to develop their skills and gain a better understanding of Down's Syndrome football.

DSActive, which also runs tennis sessions, started as a project to combat the health problems of those with DS, including obesity from lack of exercise and participation in sport, and the intention was to make football easily accessible for all abilities and ages. At school people with DS are usually excluded from being able to participate in sport, so this initiative gives them, even into adulthood, the opportunity to feel safe and comfortable and play the game they love in a competitive environment. That there are now over 40 such football teams connected to professional clubs, using top-notch facilities and coaching staff, is a mark of the value of the community these clubs are doing.

Some years ago, I met a coach from Queen's Park Rangers who had been working with young academy players, and was asked to become involved with the newly formed DS team. His first reaction, he admitted, was disappointment that he would now be working with less proficient players, which was followed by nervousness that he knew so little about disability, and particularly Down's syndrome. But once he started working with the team he became enthused by their motivation, passion and pure enjoyment. He had never enjoyed his job so much, he told me. Thanks to the dedication and professionalism of coaches like him, players began to improve, as did their grasp of tactics, positional play, and communication with one another.

Their commitment and contribution was summed up by a player from Charlton Upbeats, one of the original and most successful of the DS teams: 'They are brill, they're fantastic; they make me feel proud and lovely when I play football.' Since 2014 six adults with Down's Syndrome have completed their Level One FA coaching badges – these qualifications aren't differentiated in any way, although completion takes a little longer. Testament to the real quality exhibited by some of the players is Thomas Wade's wonder strike for Cardiff City DSActive team against Moorside Rangers in November 2012, which won Cardiff City's official Goal of the Month award.

For a number of years, the DSA ran a football tournament, the Danny Mardell Knockout Challenge, named after an East End businessman and boxer who raised money for the DSA, but died in 2005 at the age of 43. (His son Danny 'The Boss' Mardell Jr, who has Down's, attended all his dad's fights. After his father's death, his mother, Carol, ensured Danny Jr got involved in boxing, and he is now following in his father's footsteps as an amateur boxer.)

It was at one of these tournaments in 2008 that our family first met Kevin Kilbane. Daniel played in one of the five-a-side teams for the DSA, and at the time declared it one of the most amazing experiences of his life: 'I was playing on the pitch at Upton Park in the same team as Sophie, a girl with Down's, and Kevin Kilbane, an international footballer – it was pretty surreal.' Kevin, who played 110 times for the Republic of Ireland, has since retired and is now a BBC television and radio pundit. He has two daughters, one of whom, Elsie, has Down's syndrome, and he is a patron of the DSA. Kevin and I worked together on his autobiography, *Killa*, and he has become a close friend.

At Spurs v West Ham game at White Hart Lane in February 2015 a disturbing incident occurred in which we became involved. I was at the game with Daniel, and we thought we could hear thousands of West Ham fans, in the opposite corner of the ground from us, singing a derogatory song about the Spurs and England centre-forward, Harry Kane. The home supporters' chant of 'Harry Kane, he's one of our own, he's one of our own' had been transformed by the away fans into, 'Harry Kane, talks like a mong, and plays like one too.'

When we got home, Daniel decided we couldn't ignore this. The chant might be adopted by supporters from other clubs and be sung throughout the land. Daniel emailed his old coach Troy Townsend (father of Crystal Palace and England's Andros Townsend) at the Kick It Out campaign. Troy immediately contacted the Football Association, who promised a thorough investigation. I tweeted about the chant, Kevin Kilbane retweeted, and then he gave an interview to Colin Young at the *Daily Mail*, in which he said that

> like racist or homophobic chanting, it is intended to cause offence. I want to be able to take my kids to football matches, and when Elsie gets older she will understand about her condition, and I would not want her to hear that kind of chanting. . . this is a wider society problem, not just a problem with football – schoolchildren still insult each other with the word 'Mong' – and idiots are using football as a tool to show their ignorance and discrimination. I have spoken to the FA, and they have assured me

they will investigate it thoroughly. In all my time playing and watching football I have never heard this before. Hopefully we can do something to make sure it isn't again, and this awful chant does not spread.

The next morning all hell had let loose, and the story was the first item on *5 Live News*. Kevin rang me to say he had never received such abuse from football supporters, who had accused him of all sorts of heinous crimes against the free speech of football fans. He had been asked to do lots of interviews about the incident, and had decided to be interviewed by Dan Walker on BBC Radio 5 Live. Kevin, who is a great ambassador for the Down's community, was very articulate and calm, and explained how sad he was on behalf of Elsie. He also made it clear that this was not just an issue involving West Ham – it wasn't even just a football issue: it was societal.

In the meantime, I was receiving some trolling on Twitter, including one tweet from a Fleetwood Town 'Ultra' (yes, there is such a person), which read, 'You idiot - a mong is short for mongrel, which is type of dog.' Where to start? I didn't.

The West Ham hierarchy, however, behaved impeccably, immediately issuing an apology on behalf of their fans, and inviting Kevin to the club to discuss the matter. Fortunately, this abusive chant hasn't been heard since.

Footballers tend to get a bad press, and there are indeed regular stories of boorish behaviour by overpaid professionals. Some of it is, of course, warranted, but there are many players that undertake charity work, which often goes unreported. A number have their own charities, and a lot more are involved in their club's community work.

Some years ago, Daniel volunteered to coach North London

A Major Adjustment

United DS team, which he loved doing, and formed some close bonds with the players. The team was later taken over by Arsenal, and their full-back Hector Bellerin and goalkeeper Petr Cech both became involved. To celebrate World Down Syndrome day in March 2017, the Irish international Seamus Coleman spent time with the Everton Community's DS team at the club's training ground, and was genuinely touched by their skill and enthusiasm. 'You can tell they must meet up once a week, because they have the basics right, and some of the goals scored and goalkeeping was brilliant.'

His fellow Irish international, West Bromwich Albion's James McClean, discovered that a Derry football team, the Oxford Bulls, whose players all have Down's syndrome, couldn't find a team to play against. So he recruited a 'McClean Select' side to play against them. Captained by McClean himself, the team included his brother Brian, former Derry City player Vincent Sweeney, and the current Coleraine player Jordan Allan. 'Our boys were a bit starstruck when he first walked in,' said Kevin Morrison, who started the Bulls, and whose son Adam plays in it, 'but after James put them through their paces in the warm-up they were ready to take him on. . . I was delighted with the memorable experience James gave the young players. I don't think James will ever appear in a more chaotic team photo,' Kevin added, 'and yet he handled it all with such great patience and grace!'

The friendship between Jay Beatty, now aged 14, and Celtic's former centre forward Georgiou Samaras received worldwide attention in 2014 after Celtic clinched the Scottish Premiership title. Samaras plucked Jay from the crowd at Celtic's Parkhead stadium, and he became part of the victory parade. The Greek international was clearly touched by the heartfelt devotion to the club the lad from County Armagh had shown, and the genuine affection between them was extraordinarily touching. A *YouTube* video of Jay on the Celtic team bus belting out their club anthem became a huge hit, and the then manager Neil Lennon gave him his title medal.

In 2014, the Manchester City midfielder and Belgian international Kevin De Bruyne, who was the official ambassador for the Antwerp Special Olympics European Summer Games, launched a very powerful advertising campaign. He had a photograph of himself digitally altered so that his facial features took on some of the characteristics of Down's syndrome. The caption read, 'Does de Bruyne deserve fewer supporters now?' It was a very imaginative and courageous act. Rio Ferdinand had done something similar in 2003 to promote the Special Olympics.

In the summer of 1993, when Sarah was just 18 months old, I made a trip to Los Angeles. I had lived in the 'City of Angels' in the early 1980s and had a number of close friends there whom I visited regularly, but this trip was different. I was going to meet our American mentors, the Hixon family, for the first time.

Coincidentally, it transpired that at the same time as my visit their daughter Lily was participating in the Californian Special Olympics. Would I like to go to the opening ceremony with them? asked Melanie, her mother, while warning me that the experience might be a bit daunting. I said I would very much like to go, and we arranged to meet at their apartment. Ken and Melanie were incredibly welcoming, and it was wonderful to meet Lily and her 'little' brother Sam (he is now married with a child, and at 6 foot 7 inches towers over Lily).

Lily was just how Ken had described her, and she was particularly inquisitive about Sarah. I was terribly moved by her interest in my little daughter. Although they were separated by age, culture and two completely different characters, they already shared a common bond. Having a child with Down's syndrome, Ken remarked to me later, was a bit like being part of the Volkswagen Association: 'Welcome. You're now part of the club. We all have our own models of varying ages and colour, with distinctive specifications, each going at a different pace. You're going to spend a lot of time talking about your particular prototype, but you'll want to know how all the other members are getting on.'

Founded in 1968 by Eunice Kennedy Shriver, the sister of John F. and Robert Kennedy, the Special Olympics is the world's largest sports organisation for children and adults with intellectual disabilities, and provides year-round training and athletic competition for nearly six million athletes in 172 countries, as well as regular national and international events. The intention is that the competitors improve their physical fitness and motor skills, and develop greater self-confidence and a more positive self-image – but that important friendships are formed and nurtured too. Around the world millions of volunteers, acting as coaches, officials and drivers, give up their time to be part of the process of creating a greater understanding of the needs and capabilities of the learning-disabled.

Once we were inside the University of California's stadium in Westwood, I was overwhelmed. For not only were we surrounded by thousands and thousands of parents, friends, relations, volunteers and helpers, but we were also enveloped by thousands of adults and children with learning disabilities and huge numbers of them had Down's syndrome.

I was aware that Melanie was carefully watching for my reactions. She gave me an affectionate hug and asked me if I was all right. Her concern as to whether I was really ready for this experience was well founded. I thought of my small daughter back home in London and desperately wanted her to be with me.

A Level Playing Field

If she were, I felt, I could focus more clearly on Sarah as her own little being, and not have this sense of her individuality becoming enmeshed in a group identity. As several of the athletes spoke to the assembled crowd of their hopes and aspirations, not only for these games, but also for their future lives, I found it difficult to hold back the tears.

Over 20 years later, in 2015, the Special Olympics World Summer Games in Los Angeles marked the event's 14th anniversary. More than 6,500 participants with learning disabilities and around half a million spectators enjoyed nine days of competition 'full of joy and friendship'. One of the most extraordinary Special Olympians is Karen Gaffney. A swimming double gold medallist in 2001, she became the first person with Down's syndrome to complete a relay swim of the English Channel. In 2013 Karen received an honorary doctorate from the University of Portland for her work in raising awareness of the abilities of people who have Down's syndrome. She now works as an educator and inspirational speaker whose own non-profit organisation, the Karen Gaffney Foundation, is dedicated to championing full inclusion for people with Down's syndrome or other learning disabilities in families, schools, communities and the workplace.

In 2017 the Special Olympics Great Britain National Summer Games took place in Sheffield. Approximately 2,600 athletes of all abilities participated in 19 events at the steel city's impressive sporting facilities, and turning Sheffield University's student halls into a buzzing Olympic village. The immense pride that comes with winning medals and achieving personal bests was the aim, but the pure enjoyment of simply taking part, in front of sizeable crowds and proud families, created a wonderful unifying spirit.

Daniel volunteered at the event, having performed a similar role at the London 2012 Olympics and Paralympics, and described it as similarly highly charged and emotional. As a bonus, he was able to spend time with familiar old friends of Sarah's and also members of his old Clubbing Crew gang. 'The regional rivalry and competition between friends,' he reflected afterwards,

> evident from spending years dedicated to the circuit, was really something to behold. Competitors ranged from those who had to hand their false teeth over to officials before the starting gun, to a young competitor who needed a cuddly toy to help him through the pressure of the event. There was no holding back in attempts to get the whole crowd on their side. As one participant emerged onto the track and bellowed, 'Let's do this for Wales!' I asked him if he was feeling patriotic. 'No,' he responded, 'I'm feeling good!'

Coincidentally, in one of the athletics events Daniel found himself supervising Robbie, Sarah's friend from her dance and drama group. When Robbie set eyes on Daniel he greeted him with such excitement and jubilation it was as if he'd already won a medal for his Greater London team. Initially, instead of focusing and preparing for the classification race, which divided the athletes according to their abilities and was less important than those to come, Robbie, an ardent West Ham fan, was more concerned with football banter, and finding different ways of insulting Tottenham Hotspur! Undeterred by the below-par performance that predictably ensued, Robbie asked if Daniel could help again a few days later by escorting the runners to the start line for the final race. Daniel told him it shouldn't be a problem. 'What a day that'll be!' responded Robbie.

On the final day of the games, as Robbie and Daniel were taking up their respective roles before the race, Robbie spontaneously delivered a rousing and emotional speech to motivate the other three athletes. The result was a stunning victory, and gold medals all round.

Dan was incredibly impressed and touched by Robbie's commitment, competitiveness and support for his fellow athletes. He was, however, disappointed that, although the event was 'a big deal', there was very little media coverage, and he couldn't help but feel that the rest of Sheffield, let alone the rest of the country, wasn't more aware of what had taken place.

In March 2010 we had attended a reception at the House of Lords to celebrate the 40th anniversary of the DSA. There we met Simon Beresford, who in 2007, at the age of 39, had become the first person with Down's syndrome to run the London Marathon. The following year he repeated the feat, raising over £20,000 for charity. We also met Simon's running partner John Dawson, who was 68 at the time, and had put him on a strict training regime. Though the pair had run 20 miles together a few times, until the day of the Marathon itself they had never done the full distance. John was nervous, as was Simon's mother, who was anxious about how her son would manage. The only person who wasn't concerned was Simon himself. 'Not worried at all. All the people cheering me. Brilliant. Made me faster.'

Soon after Simon was born his mother had been told, 'He will be backward, but won't be a complete cabbage. He'll be able to help Dad clean the car and you do the dusting.'

17

THE PURSUIT OF 'PERFECTION'

> *Many of the defectives are utterly helpless, re-*
> *pulsive and revolting in manners. Their existence*
> *is a perpetual source of sorrow and unhappiness*
> *to their parents. In my opinion, it would be an*
> *economical and humane procedure were their*
> *very existence to be painlessly terminated.*
>
> Alfred Frank Tredgold,
> *Textbook of Mental Deficiency*, 1915

Any couple can have a baby with Down's syndrome. It occurs in families from all social, economic, cultural, religious and racial backgrounds. For some unexplained reason, an error in cell development results in 47 chromosomes instead of the normal 46. As Down's syndrome is present from the time of conception, nothing a woman does in pregnancy will influence whether or not her baby has Down's syndrome. There are no factors currently known of which could have stopped the parent giving an extra chromosome.

In 1953 Professor Jerome Lejeune became widely known as the scientist who discovered that it was an extra copy of chromosome 21 that was the cause of Down's syndrome. In recent years, however, there has been some dispute about Lejeune's discovery:

an 88-year-old paediatric cardiologist called Marthe Gautier claimed that she had done most of the experimental work that led to it. With this breakthrough came the possibility of diagnosing a whole range of genetic disorders. Ironically Lejeune, a staunch Catholic, was horrified by the advent of prenatal diagnostics, which made it possible to screen foetuses for Down's syndrome and other abnormalities, and abort those afflicted. He set out to find a scientific procedure that could prevent genetic intellectual disabilities like Down's syndrome, but also campaigned tirelessly against abortion.

The genetic imbalance that results from the additional chromosome affects both intellectual and physical development. There are about a hundred characteristic features of Down's syndrome, which may or may not present themselves in any one individual. For example, the chance of having a baby with Down's syndrome increases with the age of the parent. However, more babies with Down's are born to younger women, as the overall birth-rate is higher in this age group: in fact, 80 per cent are born to women aged 35 and younger.

Nearly 20 years ago in *A Minor Adjustment* I wrote that

> Pre-natal technology has become and continues to be more and more sophisticated, and more adept at eliminating Down's syndrome. There is no doubt that the increasing availability of tests to detect the chromosomal abnormality has influenced people, and actually feeds people's fears and prejudices. Although there is supposedly a greater consciousness about disability in general, if people constantly read about and are told of the effects to rid society of Down's syndrome, their attitudes to adults who have Down's syndrome are

unlikely to be very positive. With the advance of medical technology the number of children born with Down's syndrome is likely to fall dramatically in the coming years, until there are very few people like Sarah around. Those remaining will become incredibly isolated, and their parents are going to find it increasingly difficult to accept and cope with their disability.

The first question that some people asked Allie when told about Sarah having Down's syndrome was, 'Did you have any tests?' Allie did have a blood test which measures the levels of Alpha Feta protein and indicates certain disorders, but the result was actually more 'normal' than when she had had the same test with Daniel two years previously. We didn't request an amniocentesis (in which a sample of amniotic fluid is taken from the womb and tested) because we had no reason to believe there would be any complications with the birth of our second child – and in any case, Allie was below the age when it was offered automatically.

I now dread to think what might have happened if we had known the baby had Down's syndrome, because our prejudices and fears may well have influenced us to seriously consider a termination. Since Sarah was born in 1992, pre-natal testing has become even more geared to society's pursuit of perfection and the continuing quest to produce designer babies. This has resulted in women carrying babies with Down's being targeted by a clear agenda to rid the world of people with the syndrome. Even in the 1990s it was clear that, if a foetus was abnormal, most health professionals would expect the woman to have a termination.

But the point of testing should be to give parents all the necessary information for a decision either to prepare for the birth of your child or to terminate – not just be the precursor to an inevitable abortion. There is a difference between screening offered as a way of giving parents a choice, and Down's Syndrome being a reason to terminate. Couples who refuse pre-natal testing already often find that their decision is met with disbelief. Prospective parents are still being pressurised into termination when given a very pessimistic view of the life chances of someone with Down's syndrome. There is an assumption that parents will want a termination, and a concern that people are sometimes rushed into decisions.

In the present day the issue is even more stark. Non-Invasive prenatal testing (NIPT), a new form of screening that involves an optional blood test at around nine or ten weeks into a pregnancy, is likely to be available on the NHS from April 2018, and is approximately 99 per cent accurate for genetic conditions such as Down's, Edward's and Patau's syndromes, although women who test positively will still need to undergo an invasive amniocentesis that does carry a risk of miscarriage. While people with Down's syndrome are making great strides, and are included in society to an increasing extent, the movement to screen them out with new tests will inevitably lead to pressure to terminate pregnancies. Such an outcome is likely to have a profoundly negative impact on the DS community.

The actress and writer Sally Phillips has three sons, and her oldest, Olly, has Down's syndrome, something she and her husband didn't know until he was ten days old. His diagnosis and welcome to the world were greeted by the medics with words of warning: heart problems, a higher risk of developing leukaemia. . . 'Don't worry,' one doctor even said, 'some of them live quite as long time. . .' 'A sense of humour and dance ability were not mentioned,' says Sally.

It wasn't long before I'd begun to feel like a fraud. I was still getting lots of head tilts and sympathy, but my life hadn't been ruined at all. Far from it. It was different, that's all. More challenges, but a lot more laughter, too... All we can know for sure about a baby born with Down's syndrome today is that this generation will definitely exceed the expectations of the last. I was told Olly, now aged 13, might not walk. He walks, runs, swims and rides a bike. I was told he might not talk. He recites poetry, he acts, he plays the piano.

Far from Olly being a 'problem', a 'challenge', Sally describes him as 'a blessing': 'People with Down's syndrome rejoice in simply being alive. They are irrepressible, full of enjoyment. In all senses, they have something extra – not something less.'

In autumn 2016 a BBC2 documentary, *A World without Down's Syndrome*, presented by Sally, examined whether NIPT will eventually eradicate Down's syndrome.

I started making my documentary because I don't feel that Down's syndrome is a disability so severe that it warrants such huge government investment in so many state-of-the art tests. However, while making the documentary I heard many, many stories of women being pressurised by medical professionals to screen, and even to terminate. We have the most expensive state-of-the-art Down's syndrome detection test, and the ability to terminate right up until birth.

The Pursuit of 'Perfection'

(Abortion is legal up to 24 weeks, but the 1967 Act extends the limit until birth if there is significant risk of the baby having serious disabilities.)

In the documentary, Sally visited Iceland, where the introduction of the test has meant that 100 per cent of Down's syndrome pregnancies are terminated. She interviewed Professor Kypros Nicolaides of King's College Hospital, a veteran proponent of pre-natal screening, who was quoted as saying that 'for some people having a baby with Down's is an intolerable event . . . it is a burden that goes on for a long time.' And Professor Lynn Chitty, told by Sally Phillips that her son Olly was aged 11, responded, 'He's likely to outlive you. What does that prospect hold for you?'

The programme generated huge interest and received much media coverage, and soon after it was aired, an old schoolmate of mine, Jonathan Romain, now a rabbi, appeared on BBC's *Sunday Morning Live* to discuss NIPT and the documentary. I was astonished by some of his assertions, which propagated the myths about Down's. 'They may have a happy household to begin with,' he claimed, 'but eventually they will have to give up that child to a care institution and worry themselves about not being able to visit.' He also questioned, on moral grounds, 'the point of bringing into the world a child, an adult, that cannot sustain itself, that will never be able to live independently?' Even more worrying was the revelation that, as a community leader, he had been involved in counselling parents: I was concerned that someone in such a role didn't have what I would consider a more balanced and knowledgeable view of the condition.

I had always admired Jonathan and was surprised by his attitude. So I wrote to him.

I don't take issue with your views on termination and a woman's right to choose. As far as I'm concerned, every child should be a wanted child. But this test is specifically aimed at babies with Down's syndrome. Making such an important decision must be based on correct information, and not the outmoded views that you were echoing about adults with Down's syndrome. And therein lies the crux of the matter – if future parents are told that their child will never be independent, will end up living in an institution and will be a drain on society (as you were stating), then it is inevitable that they will be influenced in their decision about whether to keep their child with DS or whether to terminate. Sarah isn't unique in her abilities. She has many friends who are similarly independent, and are by no means the individuals that society likes to stereotype. This is because they have been given the opportunities that their predecessors weren't afforded. They have changed people's attitudes. If future parents are given this sort of information, do you not think that this would make a huge difference to their decision?

Jonathan wrote back to me apologising for any distress that I might have felt, but failed to address my principal points, and his TV appearance and opinions elicited a strong response on social media from the DS community – a radical and vocal group, strengthened by a mutual resolve and support, and something Allie and I would have loved to have had during Sarah's early years.

A much angrier reaction had resulted a couple of years earlier when the geneticist Richard Dawkins created a 'Twitterstorm' by writing that it would be immoral to carry on with a pregnancy if the mother knew the foetus had Down's syndrome: 'Abort it and try again. It would be immoral to bring it into the world if you have the choice.'

In the *Spectator* Simon Barnes, *The Times* columnist and former chief sports writer, responded on behalf of his teenage son, Eddie, who has Down's. 'If we are going to be logical, then we need to do something about old people, about all people with serious illnesses, about all low-achievers – why pick on kids like Eddie?'

Dawkins never retracted his opinion, but added that not aborting the child is 'immoral' from the point of view of the child's own welfare. 'In other words', Simon Barnes retorted, 'a foetus with Down's is better off unborn.

> Logical inference: a person with Down's syndrome is better off dead. Dawkins doesn't know what it's like to be dead, and he doesn't know what it's like to have Down's syndrome, so I'm not convinced he has a valid argument here. Eddie will make people more generous, make them behave better towards other people with problems, make them think about such people in a better way. He will make people fractionally gentler and fractionally kinder. That doesn't seem to me a negligible contribution to society; many people do less. . . Dawkins implies that both society and Eddie would be better if Eddie did not exist . . . if we distil everything that matters down to its last brutal reductionist essence, what are we left with? Eddie's job in this world is to love and to be loved.

A Major Adjustment

In June 2016, alongside parents and professionals, I took part in a Nuffield Council Bio Ethics conference on the implications of NIPT for Down's syndrome and other genetic conditions. I am not against abortion, and would not like to ally myself with the pro-life lobby, but I am concerned that parents are still making decisions without knowing all the facts about Down's syndrome. Let's face it, if you are told that your baby may never walk, talk, read and write, may suffer a heart defect and be at higher risk of leukaemia and later Alzheimer's, and that he or she is destined for an unfulfilled, unhappy life, then it is likely you will choose not to continue the pregnancy. The choice must be informed – made from knowledge not ignorance – and all aspects of the positive alternative to termination must be discussed.

Information is the key element to this process, and parents must be given realistic, balanced data which is not based on ignorance and prejudice. The material in patient leaflets can be inconsistent, and some is inaccurate and out of date. Women need to be provided with truthful information on the spectrum of Down's, not just the worst-case scenario. The DSA's Tell It Right, Start It Right campaign developed information packs and resources to distribute to universities to train lecturers and health professionals involved in pre-natal screening.

In fact, the introduction of NIPT could be an opportunity to improve training and education in this field. There is also a need for good follow-up support for patients after they have had NIPT. National standards for midwives are needed, and the training of midwives involved in providing pre-natal screening is vital. Following a diagnosis face-to-face counselling with a trained person is important, especially if NIPT starts becoming available on the NHS.

There is also the question of how much money the NHS is

spending on screening, and whether some of this huge sum could be better spent on medical research, training, or more resources and facilities for those with Down's syndrome who actually exist. One might hope that we could try and maximise the potential of children and adults with Down's syndrome, rather than weed them out and destroy them before they are born.

The fiscal argument or 'cost- benefit analysis' does have a large influence on the way forward for the medical profession, particularly at this time when the NHS is desperately short of funding. Cuts in public-service spending have been particularly malevolent in recent years in regard to the incapacitated, and there exists a discriminatory ideology that disabled people dependent on state benefits are a costly burden to the state. The market economy distinguishes between 'productive and unproductive' citizens, and there is the real possibility that people who choose to bear disabled children will be considered selfish, deluded or irresponsible.

In response to NIPT, some Down's advocates formed *Don't Screen Us Out*, a campaign calling on the government to halt the implementation of cell-free DNA screening. It quoted a UNESCO report's warning that 'the potential ethical disadvantages of NIPT can be summarised as routinisation and institutionalisation of the choice of not giving birth to an ill or disabled child.'

As part of the Nuffield Council's BioEthics initiative that included the conference I attended, Mencap was commissioned to consult the views of adults with Down's syndrome on NIPT. I really wasn't sure about this – I understood the need to be inclusive, but I couldn't see what would be gained. Seven individuals participated, and the results were hardly surprising: the main conclusion was that the contributors were left questioning the value of their lives. This was an extremely complicated issue, and would need to be handled very sensitively. We asked Sarah – somewhat tentatively, as we knew it could upset her – what she thought about people with Down's syndrome not being born, and her reply was brief and to the point: 'That's not right.'

Each year about 750 babies are born with Down's syndrome – about one in every 1,000 births – and there are an estimated 30,000 people with Down's syndrome living in the United Kingdom. There is a high risk that NIPT will decrease the birth rate of people with Down's Syndrome by, it is predicted, identifying nearly 200 more foetuses as Down's each year – which, in the current climate, may well result in more women feeling pressured to make a choice to terminate. An overall decline of DS births by 13 per cent would lead, it is forecast, to a corresponding reduction in the number of people in the UK with the condition.

In countries where Down's syndrome screening has been standard for years, termination rates stand at almost 100%. Hayley Goleniowska is an extraordinary advocate for the Down's community whose energy and commitment to 'the cause' is inspirational. 'If parents are rushed into terminations,' she has written,

> or asked repeatedly if they would like to end their pregnancies, then we are certainly sending out the message that some lives are worth a great deal less than others. When screening becomes standard, and truly informed consent is not sought from prospective parents along with unbiased genetic counselling, then termination becomes the only assumed route. I would love to see Learning Disability nurses involved at precisely this stage.

In the UK, 92 per cent of pregnancies where Down's is detected are terminated, which rather adds weight to the argument that testing is primarily made available for the purposes of eradication. It is also true that fewer people with Down's syndrome in the population will lead to a de-skilling of the healthcare workforce, decreased social understanding of the condition, increased stigma, and feelings of isolation and exclusion among people who do have Down's syndrome. And those that escape the cull are much more likely to be discriminated against, and will be isolated and alienated.

The principal conclusion of the Nuffield Council's BioEthics conference was that

> *Women and couples should be able to access NIPT to enable them to find out, if they wish, whether their foetus has a significant medical condition or impairment, but only within an environment that enables them to make autonomous, informed choices, and when the potential wider harms of NIPT are minimised.*

The debate about NIPT can be reduced to individual choice but, taken collectively, it could be thought to have eugenic consequences. It may be hugely emotive to liken NIPT to 'a tool for eugenics', but there is no doubt that specific groups are being targeted, and there is a Darwinian element. It was, in fact, Darwin's theory of 'survival of the fittest' that his cousin Sir Francis Galton was led to apply to ethnicity in humans. Galton coined the term 'eugenics' in 1869, writes Joanna Ryan in *The Politics of Mental Handicap*, describing its purpose as 'to produce a highly gifted race of men by judicious marriages during several consecutive generations'. He defined two types of eugenics: 'positive eugenics' was the preferential breeding of superior individuals to improve the genetic stock of the human race; 'negative eugenics' was the discouragement or prohibition of reproduction by individuals thought to have inferior genes.

This notion of eugenics directly influenced the Aryan-race theory of the Nazis. Philip Bouhler was an early member of the Nazi party who was elected to the Reichstag in 1933 and in the following year became Munich's head of the police and subsequently Hitler's chief of chancellery, with access to Hitler's mail. In early 1939, a letter from the father of a blind and 'mentally disabled' five-month-old baby, Gerhard Kretschmar, asked the Nazi leader if he could arrange for his child to be 'put to sleep'. Bouhler offered to take over the matter and Hitler, not a details man, agreed.

The baby is believed to have been given a lethal drug, causing unconsciousness and death several days later. Gerhard's cause of death was recorded as 'heart failure'. The case was to provide the catalyst for Bouhler to authorise a strategy that would extend to German physicians the authority to provide a 'mercy death' to selected children within days of their birth. In August 1939 the Interior Ministry issued a decree ordering the systematic annihilation of mentally and physically disabled new-born children – those suspected of being 'afflicted' with idiocy and Mongolism, and malformations of all kinds, particularly the absence of limbs, severe midline defects of the head and spine, and cerebral palsy.

The euthanasia programme was code-named T4, after its street address in Berlin. The Kretschmars had wanted their son dead, but most of the other disabled children were forcibly taken from their parents to be killed. Within months it wasn't just babies that were murdered. Children were taken into local hospitals and killed by lethal injections, although their deaths were recorded as having general weakness or measles. Between 1939 and 1945 nearly 25,000 children with disabilities were killed in Germany and occupied territories. At least 300,000 with disabilities were exterminated in 'mercy killings' as part of the T4 programme.

Hundreds of hospitals, asylums and clinics took part in the Third Reich's programme to wipe out the lives of people described as 'life unworthy as life'. They were systematically incarcerated, segregated and then drugged, gassed or starved. Importantly, this was driven not just by dogma and a philosophical agenda, but also by an economic imperative. The cost of keeping an 'incurable idiot' in an increasingly market-led economy was considered a waste of money.

Within sight of one such institution, Sonnenstein, near Dresden, where nearly 14,000 'mentally retarded' people were gassed and cremated, Sarah's grandmother, Ursula, was living with her sister, Luise, and their parents. I cannot help but think what would have happened to Sarah if she had been born in Germany during that period. As a 'mental defective', or as 'life unworthy of life', would she have been part of the children's euthanasia programme, or would she somehow have survived this only to become another Jewish victim of the Final Solution?

There are between 4,000 and 6,000 diagnosed genetic disorders. It is estimated that 1 in 25 children is affected by such conditions, and so 30,000 babies and children are newly diagnosed in the UK each year. Genetic engineering may enable us to discover and counteract human diseases and disabilities that are caused by a single gene or set of genes. Genetic links have already been established with many disorders and, as studies and further genetic forays become more refined, it can't be long before we might be able to decide that we don't want a deaf baby, a blind baby, a baby that might grow up to be fat or bald, or one of those considered to be a drain on our medical resources such as alcoholics and smokers. Let's stamp out anyone who isn't 'normal', or who might be proved to be 'unproductive'. Take the notion to extremes, and one day, on some kind of genetic menu, we will be able to select academic ability, the colour of our offspring's hair and eyes, and with or without freckles.

I do not believe that Down's syndrome should be a sole reason for termination. No pre-natal tests can predict how able or disabled a child will turn out to be or what these children can eventually achieve. Most importantly, the tests cannot predict the quality of life. Society is obsessed with the idea that we should all conform to the notion of 'normality', but, instead of trying to create a world where anything unconventional is looked upon with suspicion and fear, we should be trying to accept people's individuality, and welcome those who are different.

I object to the assumption that any child who is not 'perfect' will not be wanted, and echo the words of Sally Phillips: 'If we deny someone the chance to be born because we've already decided they won't meet some predetermined measure of status or achievement, then we've seriously failed to grasp what it is to be human.' The *Guardian* journalist Frances Ryan encapsulated the debate nicely: 'Having a disabled child is said to be a tragedy or an inconvenience that should always be avoided, while women who do choose to abort a foetus with abnormalities are vilified as shallow and selfish. . . neither is accurate.'

The consequence of the introduction of NIPT, it is clear to me – whether intended or not – will be that the weight of choice will be different, and in practice women and their partners will find themselves having to proactively choose to have a child with Down's syndrome. There is likely to be stigma attached to the women who choose not to test. To avoid this, Rebecca Bennett,

The Pursuit of 'Perfection'

Professor of Ethics at the University of Manchester, has argued for a policy of voluntary non-directive testing:

> Our current 'opt-out' screening practice for Down's in pregnancy already entails an element of coercion, and sends the message that it is recommended. Offering screening and testing for Down's is important, but it should be offered without pressure to accept.

In 2017, Ali Craft and his wife Jennifer (Jen) found out that the baby they were expecting after an initial blood test and amniocentesis had Down's syndrome. There was never, at any point, a thought that they would terminate, and they really wanted to know the diagnosis in order to prepare for the baby. Jen initially announced the news on Facebook so that friends and family would be aware of their situation – this method saved lots of telephone calls and conversations and having to explain hundreds of times about how they felt. This is Jen's post:

> Today we found out that our child has Down's syndrome. A shock that I'm not sure I've fully absorbed, or I'm not sure if I ever will. I'm not ready to look reality in the face just yet – it would find me screaming at it and calling it a fucker. And yet life is like that sometimes – a right fucker, it sneaks behind your back and pulls you down a different path while you were making other plans. This is not what we had planned, for our baby or, if I'm selfish, for me and my husband.
>
> I don't want to look at support groups or blogs or articles that I'll read too much into and realise how

difficult life will be for my child, how hard to make sense of the world and their place in it. But I have seen my child, dancing on a monitor (three times now, you're lucky if you have something a bit left-field going on with your child) – this little one won't sit still, they are moving, their heart is beating, they are mine.

A child who seems to love life, they're not aware of our sleepless nights, or the tears I've shed as I've waited for the results, or the dark thought that it might be easier if they just slipped away after the shock of the news. This is a child that we wanted, that brought joy with the news of their impending arrival, a child that will be born into a huge and loving family and a strong home. I will mourn the life that we planned but, as a good friend told me, breaking down or cracking up isn't an option. I will look forward to the life that we have, to our new family – my little one's path will be more difficult than I would ever have hoped, but I am tiny Craft's mother, I will light the way as best I can. I will fight for you, little one, your life won't be easy, but you couldn't have picked a better bunch of people to have in your corner, I will love you, so much.

He husband Ali's post soon followed.

For those who haven't seen Jennifer's post (and she puts it far better than I ever could), we have just found out that our baby has Down's. The only reason I know we can do this is because of the support of our amazing family and friends, and my God are we going to need you now!

This child is going to be born into an amazingly supportive family that I have the pleasure of being born and married into, and we will do this together. This may not be what we expected, but it is going to be our family, and I'm sure that in the coming years we won't be able to imagine life any different. More than anything, I know that my wife is incredible, and our family may be a bit different, but it's going to be amazing.

The reaction from their friends and family was immediately supportive. Ali and Jen were convinced they were doing the right thing and had made the correct decision, and were also helped by the medical staff they dealt with, who never put any pressure on them to have a termination or to make them feel guilty.

Alice Hope Craft was born on 11 November 2017, is in good health, and the family are all very happy together.

At the end of October 2017, Sarah was staying with us, having danced the previous night away at a friend's wedding, and, because she needed to be at work early the next morning and hates the thought of being late, Allie offered to drive her into town. On her way home, Allie tuned in to Radio 4's *Sunday* programme. Kári Stefánsson, one of the world's leading geneticists, who had featured in *A World Without Down's Syndrome*, was being interviewed. 'When I was at medical school 40 years ago,' he was saying, 'one of the goals of obstetrics and gynaecologists was to screen in such a way that Down's syndrome could be eradicated. Now, 40 years later, here we are in Iceland, where no children are born with Down's syndrome.'

A Major Adjustment

Allie, having just dropped Sarah off at her swanky West End hotel, was furious. So proud of her beautiful daughter's enthusiasm for the day ahead and eagerness to be independent, she had to listen to a description of a world that would deny Sarah's very existence. An outraged Allie came home absolutely fuming. 'I wanted to punch that Icelandic geneticist in his smug mush!' And Allie is not known, in these parts, or indeed anywhere, as a violent woman. . .

Although we still have a long way to go in changing society's view of the disabled, and achieving the goal of total acceptance, there is now a greater awareness of Down's syndrome. Sarah's generation is the first that has not been written off completely at birth. The tragedy is that the next generation may be written off *before* birth.

18

'I LOVE MY LIFE'

I shall be telling this with a sigh
Somewhere ages and ages hence:
Two roads diverged in a wood, and I,
I took the one less travelled by.

Robert Frost, 'The Road Not Taken'

One morning when Sarah was 14, in the wee small hours, she came downstairs, a little distressed, clutching a battered copy of *A Minor Adjustment*. The rest of the family were asleep, and I thought Sarah was too, but in fact she had been reading all about herself for the first time. When I wrote the following sentence, I hadn't ever envisaged that Sarah would be clever enough to read it, or courageous enough to confront me.

> *I was looking at my daughter – not even a day old –*
> *and wishing her dead.*

Sarah was more indignant than angry. 'I'm not happy about this, Dad.'
'What?'
'You wanted me dead.'
'Of course I didn't.'

'You wrote it!'

'Yes, but I didn't want you to suffer. . . You see, I wasn't sure . . . what was going to . . . and we didn't know you.'

This was nightmarish.

I tried to explain that, when she was first born, she had a hole in the heart. We didn't know how ill she was going to be; we didn't know whether she might ever be able to walk or talk. My description sounded hollow, and I was ashamed of what I had written, although it was how I felt at the time.

Sarah, understandably, needed much persuasion that this wasn't how I or the rest of the family now felt about her. I told her that she must know how much we all loved her, and how none of us could imagine life without her. Sarah finally went back to bed, and I hoped that I had reassured her, but I felt awful. She hasn't ever raised this again, and I think she now realises the context of those raw feelings just a few hours after she was born. If only we had known then what we know now.

One of the most difficult things about parenting a child with Down's syndrome in those days was the prospect of a very uncertain future. Although we did adapt to the philosophy of coping with Sarah stage by stage, we couldn't help thinking of how things were going to be in one, two, five, or even twenty or fifty years' time. Would she be independent? Would she work? Have relationships? Have sex? Would Sarah ever celebrate her own wedding? Could she become a mother? Develop Alzheimer's disease or leukaemia, which are more prevalent in Down's?

And now, 26 years after her dramatic birth, Sarah has answered most of those questions, and is old enough and bright enough to understand. Her arrival with a flourish and a determined expression on her kisser – 'Hello. Here I am. Deal with it' – was somewhat prescient of how her future unfolded. And, by the way, she doesn't just 'happen to have Down's syndrome', an oft-used phrase by proud parents when describing the remarkable achievements of their offspring. Sarah *has* Down's syndrome, and it has affected her throughout her life thus far, and will continue to do so. But without it neither would she be who she is – nor indeed would our family be who we are.

Sarah is very much aware about what it means to be different and to have Down's syndrome. We have always encouraged her to talk about what it is. 'I understand a bit of my disability now,' she has told us – 'I didn't before. I am normal, but I have extra chromosomes. It stops me from being like my brothers: I can't travel abroad on my own, or drive.' I did point out to her that both Daniel and Joel passed their driving tests at their first attempt some years ago and haven't driven since, for various reasons. It's not just Down's syndrome that has prevented her from taking to the road, although I must add that the world is probably a safer place without Sarah behind the wheel.

I wrote in *A Minor Adjustment* about the life-affirming effect that children and people with Down's syndrome have upon the world, but shrank from the assertion that 'every home should have one'. But it is true that Sarah and her friends have changed our lives in unimagined ways since her birth. By overcoming the pain and fear we felt at her birth we have grown, and have learned to know people truly as individuals, rather than just pay lip service to the notion. She has introduced us to a completely new world, where we have met a whole host of acquaintances, and people we just wouldn't have come across in our 'previous' lives. Even more important are the valuable, lifelong friendships we have struck up with other parents. We have also discovered deeper relationships with existing friends, and forged even closer links with our immediate family.

A Major Adjustment

Sarah has demonstrated how much someone with a learning disability can achieve with the right support and opportunities. Inevitably, great strides in awareness have been made. We have come some way from the days when people with Down's syndrome were systematically written off at birth, abused, denied a legal education and medical interventions, and had their human rights and voices ignored. But there remain difficult times and an uncertain future.

'The true measure of any society,' Mahatma Gandhi is quoted as saying, 'can be found in how it treats its most vulnerable members.' Unfortunately, the present climate doesn't make for pleasant reading. Austerity and welfare reforms have resulted in higher levels of poverty, and a reduced standard of living for disabled people. This country has never been so wealthy, and yet iniquitous spending cuts are causing untold distress, with the lives of the most vulnerable hit far harder than any other group.

A recent Mencap report on the treatment of learning-disabled hospital patients is horrifying. Deaths have also occurred at NHS assessment and treatment units for adults with learning disabilities. In July 2013 Connor Sparrowhawk, who was 18 and had learning difficulties and epilepsy, was found submerged in water at Slade House, an NHS care and assessment unit in Oxford. An inquest ruled that neglect contributed to his death, but it was only four years later that Southern Health NHS Foundation Trust, which ran the unit, admitted failings and pleaded guilty at Banbury Magistrates' Court to breaching health and safety law. 'The care Connor received was of an unacceptable standard,' said a spokesperson for the Sparrowhawk family.

> Connor's death was fully preventable . . . it has been a long and tortuous battle to get this far, and even

during the inquest the trust continued to disclose new information, including the death of another patient in the same bath in 2006. Families should not have to fight for justice and accountability from the NHS.

The current environment in the UK is such that it is the first signatory to the UN Convention on Disabled People's Rights in which the UN has found 'grave and systematic violations'. The Equality *Act of 2010* makes it unlawful to 'directly or indirectly discriminate against, harass or victimise disabled children and young people, requiring support from the welfare system', but in August 2017 the UN Committee on the Rights of Persons with Disabilities reported that the UK Government, through its welfare cuts, had created a 'human catastrophe', and was 'totally neglecting the vulnerable situation people with disabilities find themselves in'. The committee also raised concerns about 'the persisting occurring incidents of negative attitudes, stereotypes and prejudice against persons with disabilities.' In certain sections of the press the disabled are often labelled as 'scroungers' and 'benefit cheats', creating a zeitgeist of rising hostility. As a result, hate crimes against the disabled rise each year.

There is now, however, a powerful Down's lobby at work, constantly watching for any prejudice, discrimination or illegalities – thousands of wannabe Don Quixotes, on chivalrous quests, righting wrongs and bringing justice – and it no longer feels that we are still tilting at windmills. On social media the Down's syndrome community is actually quite remarkable: apart from the various professional organisations and charities that exist to help parents, the dedication of user groups, providing encouraging, positive messages, is quite humbling. When Sarah was born there were only a couple of American support groups on the internet, whereas now, what with blogs, Twitter and websites, the ether is thick with news stories, campaigns and personal accounts, all about Down's syndrome.

Meanwhile, people with Down's are increasingly achieving more, and are also more integrated than ever before. Sarah is reaping the rewards of changing attitudes and gains fought for by previous generations. 'There does still remain the inconsistencies of experience and ambiguities of feeling in having a child with Down's syndrome,' I wrote 20 years ago in *A Minor Adjustment*.

> Every day I worry about her and wish that we didn't have this extra responsibility. I wish Sarah wasn't going to have to face all these extra problems. I wish that she hadn't been born with Down's syndrome, but if she didn't have Down's syndrome she wouldn't be Sarah. I want society to accept her as she is, but I know that in her lifetime it's more likely that she will have to adapt to society first. I want her to be independent, but I want to protect her. I want her to be treated like everyone else and, unlike Blanche DuBois, I don't want her to have to depend on the kindness of strangers. Conversely, I do also want people to make allowances for her. I want her to be as bright and insightful as possible, but not enough to be aware of how society at large may perceive her. I want to accept Sarah for who she is – with all her faults and limitations – but at the same time I will also do all that I can to extend these boundaries so that she can achieve everything possible.

'I Love My Life'

Twenty years later I am aware that the adjustment is incomplete at times, and will continue to take different forms at different stages of Sarah's life. We had wondered what was going to happen to Sarah when she started to take an interest in boys (I took a heterosexual approach then, purely for convenience' sake) – and whether her affections might ever be reciprocated. That was something else we needn't have worried about. Sarah has had a few boyfriends over the years, all of whom have behaved impeccably. She has now been going out with Leon for a couple of years, and we thoroughly approve. Not only is he sweet, kind, patient and loving: more importantly he is also a Spurs fan. There is now talk of marriage, although for various reasons it is likely to be a long engagement. He is the Nathan Detroit to her Miss Adelaide.

Sarah has always amazed us with her spirit, enthusiasm and determination, whilst her capacity for warmth and honesty is profound. She has always exhibited a sensitivity and an empathetic nature. She rings at least once a day for a chat, and to see how Allie and I are. If one of the family is upset or unwell, she is invariably the one to notice and remember, and try to make things better. She judges our moods imperceptibly, and seems to have an uncanny knack of knowing when something isn't quite right.

And she has always made us laugh. She used to be absolutely hopeless at keeping secrets, and when she was about ten, I was repeating some gossip. Sarah looked worried and said, 'Sshh, Dad – remember I'm here.' Joel does a very good impersonation of a close family friend, whom we shall call Martin, and we got him to do it once for Sarah. When he had finished, she shrugged her shoulders and, unimpressed, said, 'Martin does it better.' Recently, after they'd watched the movie *Bad Mom*, which contains lots of swearing, Allie asked Sarah, 'Do you think *I'm* a Bad Mom?'

'No,' Sarah replied. 'You're fucking awesome.'

My relationship with Sarah is very special. To paraphrase the American humorist S.J. Perelman, 'I tried to resist her overtures, but she plied me with symphonies, quartets, chamber music and cantatas.' OK, I've never really tried to resist, and Kylie is more her hammer than Khachaturian, but you get the picture.

I recently told her that we would always be there to help her, we all loved her dearly, and she could ring us any time, day or night, if she needed us. She looked at me quizzically and replied, 'I know that, Dad. I love you too – but I don't *need* you.'

So, Sarah, if there is ever going to be a third book in years to come to complete a trilogy, then I want you to write it.

No . . . no, never mind – forget it. You're going to be far too busy. . .

Acknowledgements

I am most grateful to my editor, Graham Coster, for his peerless expertise, calm guidance and extraordinary efficiency. This is our fourth book together, and I hope there will be more.

I am greatly indebted to the fathers of children with Down's syndrome for their time and contributions to Chapter 9, 'Further Paterfamilias Territory', and I also wish to acknowledge that I have borrowed shamelessly from the research of Brian Stratford, Cliff Cunningham and Kieron Smith.

'Ev'ry Time We Say Goodbye': words and music by Cole Porter, ©1944 Chappell & Co. Inc. (ASCAP)

The extract on page 263 from 'The Road Not Taken' by Robert Frost is from *The Collected Poems*, published by Vintage Classics. Reproduced by permission of The Random House Group Ltd. ©2013.

Thanks also to Carol Boys, Gillian Bird, Alexa Dizon, Stuart Mills, Kate Potter, Sharon Gordon-Roberts and Veronica Mulenga at the Down's Syndrome Association, and all the staff at Foxes Academy, especially Ben Graham and Clare Walsh.

A Major Adjustment

To the following for their time, assistance and contributions: Tom Bachofner, Simon Barnes, Lucy and Otto Baxter, Anita Brady, the Cahill family, Chris Charles, Lisa Clarke, Ali and Jennifer Craft, Peter Davison, Kirstie Edwards, Steve Epstein, Blake Ezra, Fiona Yaron-Field, Angela Flowers, Liz Franks and Jason Ell, Hayley Goleniowska, Sarah Gordy, the Hardie family, Rachel Heller, the Hixons, Matthew Horsnell, Pete Houghton, Annalie Huberman, Kevin Kilbane, Grevel Lindop, Lillie Marks, Guy Milnes, Suzie Moffat, Steve Palmer, Lucy Parry, Sally Phillips, the Philpott family, Tim Reid, Paul Richards, Michel Roux Jr, Donna and Andrew Self, Hal Shinnie, Edwina Simon, Kieron Smith, Dawn Taylor, Caroline White and Aviv, Noa and Ophir Yaron.

Our friends (too many to list) and family have provided extraordinary support from the day Sarah was born, and a special mention must be made of grandmothers Jean Merriman and Ursula Wellemin.

To Daniel and Joel – not only for their treasured contributions to the book, but also for being such brilliant sons, siblings and all-round great 'lads'. (That will annoy Joel).

I am eternally grateful to Allie for her love, great support, and for being my fiercest critic. Apart from being photo editor, she was also my part-time co-author. In fact, Allie really should have a had a co-writing credit. Oh, well, I'll get her to talk to my agent . . . which reminds me: I must get an agent.

Oh, I nearly forgot . . . the person without whom this book would have been a lot of blank pages, and our lives would have been a slim volume.

Thank you, Sarah, for being you.

Select Bibliography

Bailey, Richard (ed.), *Shifting Perspectives*, BH Editions, 2012

Beaumont, Henny, *Hole in the Heart – Bringing up Beth*, Myriad Editions, 2016

Bérubé, Michael, *Life As We Know It*, Pantheon, 1996

Boston, Sarah, *Too Deep for Tears*, Pandora, 1994

Burleigh, Michael, *Death and Deliverance: Euthanasia in Germany 1900–1945*, Cambridge University Press, 1994

Cunningham, Cliff, *Down's Syndrome – An Introduction for Parents*, Souvenir Press, 1988

Donald, J. (ed.), *Uncommon Fathers: Reflections on Raising a Child with a Disability*, Woodbine House, 1995

Evans, Suzanne, *Hitler's Forgotten Victims*, Tempus, 2007

Goleniowska, Mia and Hayley, *I Love You Natty*, DownsSideup, 2014

Lewis, Sandy, *Living with Max*, Vermilion, 2008

Lott, Bret, *Jewel*, Washington Square, 1992

Merriman, Andy, *A Minor Adjustment*, Pan Macmillan, 1999

Merriman, Andy, *Tales of Normansfield*, DSA, 2007

Ryan, J. and Thomas, F., *The Politics of Mental Handicap*, Free Association Books, 1987

Selikowitz, Mark, *Down Syndrome: The Facts*, Oxford University Press, 1990

Smith, Kieron, *The Politics of Down Syndrome*, Zero, 2011

Stratford, Brian, *Down's Syndrome: Past, Present and Future*, Penguin, 1989

Stratford, Brian (ed.), *New Approaches to Down Syndrome*, Cassell, 1996

White, Caroline (author) and Sandra Isaksson (illustrator), *The Label: A Story for Families*, Ivy Press, 2016

Wright, David, *Down's – The History of a Disability*, Oxford University Press, 2011

Yaron-Field, Fiona, *Up Close – A Mother's View*, Bunker Hill, 2008